CASE STUDIES

to accompany

Clinical Manifestations
and Assessment of
RESPIRATORY DISEASE

CASE STUDIES

to accompany

Clinical Manifestations and Assessment of RESPIRATORY DISEASE

Terry Des Jardins, MEd, RRT
Director, Department of Respiratory Care
Parkland College
Champaign, Illinois

George G. Burton, MD, FACP, FCCP, FAARC
Medical Director, Respiratory Services
Kettering Medical Center
Kettering, Ohio
Clinical Professor of Medicine and Anesthesiology
Wright State University School of Medicine
Dayton, Ohio

FOURTH EDITION

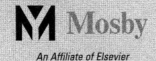
Mosby
An Affiliate of Elsevier

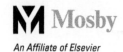

An Affiliate of Elsevier

Publishing Director: Andrew Allen
Acquisitions Editor: Karen Fabiano
Developmental Editor: Mindy Copeland
Editorial Assistant: Ellen Wurm
Project Manager: Linda McKinley
Production Editor: Kristin Hebberd
Interior/Cover Designer: Julia Ramirez
Cover Illustration: Timothy H. Phelps

4th EDITION

Copyright © 2002 by Mosby, Inc.

NOTICE

Pharmacology is an ever-changing field. Standard safety precautions must be followed, but as new research and clinical experience broaden our knowledge, changes in treatment and drug therapy may become necessary or appropriate. Readers are advised to check the most current product information provided by the manufacturer of each drug to be administered to verify the recommended dose, the method and duration of administration, and contraindications. It is the responsibility of the licensed prescriber, relying on experience and knowledge of the patient, to determine dosages and the best treatment for each individual patient. Neither the publisher nor the editor assumes any liability for any injury and/or damage to persons or property arising from this publication.

Permissions may be sought directly from Elsevier's Health Sciences Rights Department in Philadelphia, PA, USA: phone: (+1) 215 239 3804, fax: (+1) 215 239 3805, email: healthpermissions@elsevier.com. You may also complete your request on-line via the Elsevier homepage (http://www.elsevier.com), by selecting 'Customer Support' and then 'Obtaining Permissions'.

Printed in the United States of America

ISBN-13: 978-0-323-01075-7
ISBN-10: 0-323-01075-X

12   9

To all the anonymous patients who provide the foundation for the case study scenarios in this book and to our respiratory therapy students, who are always one step ahead of us.
Terry Des Jardins
George G. Burton

Preface

The delivery of effective respiratory care requires critical thinking skills. Both students and practitioners in the respiratory care profession need strong assessment skills. *Case Studies to Accompany Clinical Manifestations and Assessment of Respiratory Disease* is designed to serve the following functions:

1. Help respiratory students learn when and how to assess patients
2. Challenge practitioners to build and perfect the assessment skills they use every day in clinical practice
3. Guide managers through the successful implementation of a therapist-driven protocol (TDP) program

Two major pillars form the foundation of strong assessment skill—a knowledge base of the major respiratory diseases and competency in the performance skills of the assessment process. Before the respiratory care practitioner is permitted to work unsupervised in a TDP program, training and competency in these two areas must be attained and documented.

This workbook is designed to be used in conjunction with *Clinical Manifestations and Assessment of Respiratory Disease,* 4th edition. The case studies take the information acquired from *Clinical Manifestations* and require the user to apply it to evolving case studies that build on commonly used TDPs. By using the two books together, the reader has the opportunity to systematically gather data, formulate assessments, select appropriate treatment plans, and document all the steps involved.

Part I provides an overview of the assessment process and knowledge base needed to perform successfully in a TDP environment. Parts II through XIII present 29 case studies, each of which represents a chapter found in *Clinical Manifestations and Assessment of Respiratory Disease.* Following the case studies of six of the most commonly encountered respiratory disorders, Key Point Questions challenge the reader to pinpoint fundamental concepts related to the specific respiratory disease.

Appendix I is an answer key, including suggested responses for the case study assessment and treatment selections (subjective, objective, assessment, plans [SOAPs]), thorough and thought-provoking discussion of each case, and answers to Key Point Questions. Appendix II is an example of a respiratory assessment flow chart (SOAP) form.

Terry Des Jardins, MEd, RRT
George G. Burton, MD, FACP, FCCP, FAARC

How to Use This Book

The purposes of this book are (1) to help students or practitioners expand their knowledge base and assessment skills independently and (2) to provide instructors or managers with a tool for teaching, evaluating, and documenting the competence of their students or staff members in making assessments and treatment selections. The pages are perforated for the latter use.

Preceding the first assessment subjective, objective, assessment, plan ([SOAP])* are (1) the patient's admitting history, (2) clinical data related to the patient's initial physical examination, and (3) the specific respiratory therapy the patient is receiving. For example, the information may state the following: "An arterial blood gas was obtained while the patient was receiving 2 L/min O_2 by nasal cannula." Readers who are not satisfied with the results of a selected therapy are expected to increase or decrease the therapy or change it appropriately.

Readers are challenged to assess and treat the patients described in this book by thoroughly and systematically recording patient data. Several times within each case the reader is asked to create a problem-oriented medical record (POMR) for the patient, which includes the following information:

- The subjective and objective data collected from the patient (S-O)
- An assessment based on the subjective and objective data (A)
- The treatment plan (with measurable outcomes; P)

One of the most common POMR methods is the formulation of a SOAP progress note. SOAP is an acronym for the following four specific aspects of charting a patient's condition:

S: Subjective information refers to perceptions provided by the patient about his or her feelings, concerns, or sensations, as follows:
- "I coughed hard all night long."
- "My chest feels very tight."

Only the patient can provide subjective information. A comatose, intubated patient on a mechanical ventilator therefore cannot provide subjective data.

---

*Weed LL: Medical record, medical education, and patient care: the problem-oriented record as a basic tool, Cleveland, Ohio, 1971, Case Western Reserve University Press.
All the assessment answers in Appendix I are presented in the SOAP format: subjective, objective, assessment, plan (see Fig. 1-4). For a more in-depth discussion of the SOAP format, see Des Jardins T, Burton GG: Clinical manifestations and assessment of respiratory disease, ed 4, St Louis, 2002, Mosby.

O: Objective information includes the data the respiratory care practitioner can measure, factually describe, or obtain from other clinical reports or test results. Objective data include the following:

- Heart rate
- Respiratory rate
- Blood pressure
- Temperature
- Breath sounds
- Cough effort
- Sputum production (volume, consistency, color, and odor)
- Arterial blood gas and pulse oximetry data
- Pulmonary function study results
- X-ray findings
- Hemodynamic data
- Chemistry results

A: Assessment refers to the practitioner's professional conclusion about what is the "cause" and severity of the subjective and objective data. In a patient with a respiratory disorder the cause is most commonly due to a specific anatomic alteration of the lung. The assessment is the specific reason "why" the respiratory care practitioner is working with the patient. For example, the presence of wheezing would be objective data (the clinical indicator) to verify the assessment (the cause) of bronchial smooth muscle constriction; arterial blood gases—pH 7.18, $Paco_2$ 80 mm Hg, HCO_3^- 29 mmol/L, and Pao_2 54 mm Hg—would be the objective data to verify the assessment of acute ventilatory failure with moderate hypoxemia; or the presence of rhonchi would be a clinical indication verifying the assessment of secretions in the large airways.

P: Plan is the therapeutic procedure(s) selected to remedy the cause identified in the assessment that is responsible for the subjective and objective data. For example, an assessment of bronchial smooth muscle constriction would justify the administration of a bronchodilator; the assessment of acute ventilatory failure would justify mechanical ventilation.

SOAP Example

A 26-year-old man arrived in the emergency room with a severe asthmatic episode. On observation, his arms were fixed to the bedrails; he was using his accessory muscles of inspiration; and he was pursed-lip breathing. The patient stated, "It feels like someone is standing on my chest. I just can't seem to take a deep breath." His heart rate was 111 bpm, blood pressure 170/110, and respiratory rate 28/min and shallow. Hyperresonant notes were produced on percussion. Auscultation revealed expiratory wheezing and rhonchi bilaterally. His chest x-ray revealed a severely depressed diaphragm and alveolar hyperinflation. His peak expiratory flow rate (PEFR) was 165 L/min. Although his cough effort was weak, he produced a large amount of thick, white sputum. His arterial blood gases (on room air) were as follows: pH 7.27, $Paco_2$ 62 mm Hg, HCO_3^- 25 mmol/L, and Pao_2 49 mm Hg.

S: "It feels like someone is standing on my chest. I can't take a deep breath."

O: Use of accessory muscles of inspiration; pursed-lip breathing; hyperresonance; expiratory wheezing; depressed diaphragm and alveolar hyperinflation; PEFR 165; weak cough; large amount of thick, white sputum; pH 7.27; $Paco_2$ 62; HCO_3^- 25; Pao_2 49

A: Bronchospasm
- Hyperinflation
- Poor ability to mobilize thick secretions
- Acute ventilatory failure with severe hypoxemia

P: Initiate bronchodilator therapy per protocol; bronchial hygiene therapy protocol; and mechanical ventilation per protocol. Check ABGs q30min.

After the treatment has been administered, another abbreviated SOAP note should be made to determine whether the treatment plan needs to be "up-regulated" or "down-regulated." Because of the nature of this book, the patient does not always respond well to therapy–even when the appropriate therapy or follow-up therapy has been selected. For this reason, each case is discussed in detail (see Appendix I), and readers are further encouraged to discuss their treatment selections and possible patient outcomes with fellow students or therapists and with instructors or managers.

FOR USE IN AN ACADEMIC SETTING

Even with a strong knowledge base of the major respiratory disorders, the student needs time and practice to carry out the actual assessment process. Initially, this process should be done in a controlled classroom environment. Ideally these sessions should be conducted after (or during) the presentation of each major respiratory disorder in the curriculum.

During these practice sessions, students may work individually or in small groups on the cases presented in this book. The authors recommend that each student or a representative from each group present the assessment(s) and treatment selection(s) to the rest of the class on a chalkboard or overhead projector. For example, all the group representatives could go to the chalkboard and write their assessment and treatment selections on the board.

The instructor also should ask the students to indicate (1) which specific treatment they have selected under a particular treatment protocol category (for example, incentive spirometry or continuous positive airway pressure under the Hyperinflation Therapy Protocol) and (2) the intensity with which it is to be administered (for example, treatment frequency bid or qid). This activity often stimulates both the students and the instructor to identify certain problems and discuss acceptable assessments and treatment selections. Instructors who wish to present the cases in this book as testing exercises, rather than as review or homework, should remove the perforated pages in Appendix I on the first day of class.

FOR USE IN A CLINICAL SETTING

All respiratory students and hospital staff members should at some time be required to put into writing (for documentation purposes) their success with several different patient assessment exercises, which could include the following:

1. Work through the cases in this book, disease by disease, without the answers in Appendix I, which are perforated. Turn in "SOAPed" cases to the clinical instructor or hospital supervisor.
2. Critically review and assess a past case. Did respiratory care do a good job? Did it do a bad job? Why or why not?
3. Write an assessment and treatment plan for several different patients throughout the hospital. A competent therapist will not need more than 10 or 15 minutes per case to complete this task.
4. Spend an entire day with the medical director. The student may be asked by the physician to provide a written assessment of and treatment plan for numerous patients around the hospital.

Ideally, two or more qualified assess-and-treat respiratory therapists should be involved in the evaluation and check-off process of respiratory clinical staff members (working to prove and document competency) or respiratory students (working on their clinical requirements). These qualified therapists could include the *Assessment* course instructor, key clinical instructors, respiratory care department heads, supervisors, or medical directors.

An assessment and treatment (SOAP) form (see Fig. 1-4 and Appendix II) is often helpful in both the classroom and the clinical setting in the rapid collection and systematic organization of important clinical data, the formulation of an assessment, and the development of a treatment plan. The SOAP form provided also may serve as a final testing tool and be placed on file for documentation, along with the "SOAPed" cases from this book. Such documentation should be updated periodically to validate the retention of assessment skills.

KEY POINTS FOR KEY DISEASES

A special feature–Key Point Questions–can help enhance the reader's knowledge of those respiratory disorders most frequently encountered in the clinical setting: chronic bronchitis, asthma, pneumonia, pulmonary edema, adult respiratory distress syndrome, and postoperative atelectasis. The points that should be known and understood about these diseases are presented in the Key Point Questions. The question format, which is used to develop the critical-thinking ability every respiratory care practitioner should use in assessment and treatment selection, appears in the following sequence:

1. *Basic Concept Formation* questions cover common knowledge and common-sense information about the disorder, helping to establish the typical lay person's perception of the disorder. Questions in this section might include the following in a patient with asthma: What are the general *anatomic alterations of the lungs* associated with the disorder (e.g., bronchospasm)? What are the common *causes* of the disorder (e.g., allergy to cat hair)? A person who has a brother or sister with asthma, for example, probably has more background knowledge about the disorder than the general public would have. The idea behind categorizing some concepts as basic is first to *recognize* the concepts and then to use them as a framework from which to build the database in the next section.

2. *Database Formation* questions cover new and in-depth concepts the respiratory care practitioner should know and understand regarding the interrelationships of the *anatomic alterations of the lungs, pathophysiologic mechanisms, clinical manifestations,* and *treatment modalities.* Questions in this section might include the following: What is your image or vision of the anatomic alterations of the lungs associated with the respiratory disorder? (See Fig. 1-14 for an illustration of a three-component model of a prototype airway. Therapy may be directed to any or all components.) Which pathophysiologic mechanisms are commonly activated as a result of the anatomic alterations of the lungs? Which clinical manifestations are commonly activated as a result of the respiratory disorder?

3. *Assessment* questions cover information needed to assess and treat a patient with this disorder effectively. This section provides a more in-depth review of the clinical data presented in the case study, which in turn reflects the specific anatomic alterations of the lungs and the pathophysiologic mechanisms caused by the respiratory disorder. This section also looks at the issue of severity rating of the clinical manifestations presented. Questions in this section

might include the following: In this case, which clinical manifestations support your assessment as to (1) your image of the *anatomic alterations* of the lungs and (2) the *pathophysiologic* mechanisms activated? Which specific clinical manifestations do you feel were the most important clinical indicators of the severity of the disorder?

4. *Application* questions cover those actions the therapist can take to treat the patient's specific, identified problems. This section looks at the selection of treatment protocols and modalities that will be the most effective in correcting or offsetting clinical manifestations caused by the anatomic alterations and pathophysiologic mechanisms associated with the disorder. Questions in this section might include the following: Based on the clinical data and your assessments, which treatment protocols are indicated in treating the problems identified? What are the advantages and disadvantages of the treatment modalities selected?

5. *Evaluation* questions cover the outcome analysis. This section includes the analysis of the way in which the patient is responding to treatment. Questions in this section might include the following: What are the expected outcomes of each of the treatment protocols you selected? What should be monitored to determine how the patient is reponding to the treatment modalities selected?

6. *Boundary Awareness* questions cover when and whom the practitioners should ask for help. Questions in this section might include the following: What signs indicate the patient's condition is approaching unsafe boundaries? At what point should a supervisor be asked to help? At what point should the patient's physician be called?

After studying the Key Point Questions and answers, the reader should be able to comfortably answer questions about the disorder in general and the case in particular.

Contents

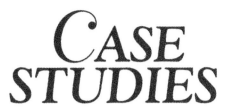

CASE
STUDIES

to accompany

Clinical Manifestations
and Assessment of
Respiratory Disease

PART I

Introduction

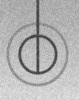

The Therapist-Driven Protocol Program and the Role of the Respiratory Practitioner

Therapist-driven protocols (TDPs) (also known as *patient-driven respiratory care protocols, respiratory assess and treat protocols,* and *respiratory consult services)* have emerged as an integral part of respiratory care health services. Regardless of the specific term or phrase used, all respiratory protocols in a good TDP program are based on the *Clinical Practice Guidelines* recently developed by the American Association for Respiratory Care (AARC).

Respiratory TDPs provide much-needed flexibility for the administration of therapeutic care to patients. For example, protocols give the respiratory care practitioner specific authority to start, increase, decrease, and discontinue respiratory therapy on a moment-to-moment, hour-to-hour, or shift-by-shift basis after the protocol has been ordered by the attending physician. TDPs increase the quality of respiratory care by virtue of the fact that the therapy can be quickly modified in response to the specific and immediate needs of the patient. According to the American College of Chest Physicians, respiratory care protocols are defined as follows:

> ... patient care plans which are initiated and implemented by credentialed respiratory care workers. These plans are designed and developed with input from physicians, and are approved for use by the medical staff and the governing body of the hospitals in which they are used. They share in common extreme reliance on assessment and evaluation skills. Protocols are by their nature dynamic and flexible, allowing up- or down-regulation of intensity of respiratory services. Protocols allow the respiratory care practitioner authority to evaluate the patient, initiate care, to adjust, discontinue, or restart respiratory care procedures on a shift-by-shift, or hour-to-hour basis once the protocol is ordered by the physician. They must contain clear strategies for various therapeutic interventions, while avoiding any misconception that they infringe on the practice of medicine.

Recent studies have shown that when respiratory care protocols are followed correctly, significant improvements are seen in respiratory care outcomes and cost savings. *The essential components of a good TDP program, however, do not come easy.* This is because a strong TDP program promises that the respiratory practitioner identified as TDP "safe and ready" is qualified to (1) systematically collect the appropriate clinical data, (2) formulate a uniform and accurate assessment, and (3) select a uniform and optimal treatment within the limits set by the protocol (Fig. 1-1). These qualifications take a lot of training, practice, and time to meet.

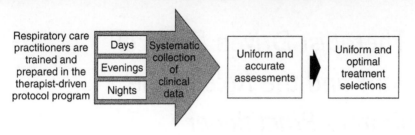

Fig. 1-1 The promise of a good TDP program.

ESSENTIALS OF A GOOD THERAPIST-DRIVEN PROTOCOL PROGRAM

As illustrated in the overview of a good TDP program in Fig. 1-2, the implementation of every respiratory care plan must be directly linked to (1) a physician's order, (2) the identification and documentation of specific clinical manifestations (obtained from both the patient's chart and physical examination), (3) a respiratory assessment and severity assessment, (4) a treatment selection that is both helpful and cost efficient, and (5) the re-evaluation of the patient's response to the treatment. This step-by-step process mandates that the respiratory care practitioner have a strong knowledge base of the major respiratory disorders and be competent in the actual assessment process.

The Knowledge and Skills Base

As shown in Fig. 1-3, the essential knowledge base includes (1) the anatomic alterations of the lungs caused by common respiratory disorders, (2) the major pathophysiologic mechanisms activated throughout the respiratory system as a result of the anatomic alterations, (3) the common clinical manifestations that develop, and (4) the treatment modalities used to correct them. Each respiratory disease chapter presented in this workbook provides these four essential knowledge components necessary for TDP work. The respiratory care practitioner should know and understand why certain and expected clinical manifestations appear in certain respiratory disorders. This knowledge base enhances the assessment and treatment selection process.

The Assessment Process

The respiratory care practitioner with good assessment skills also must be competent in performing the actual assessment process. This means the practitioner can (1) quickly and systematically gather the important clinical manifestations demonstrated by the patient from both the patient's chart and physical examination, (2) formulate an accurate assessment of the clinical data (i.e., identify the *cause* and *severity* of the data), (3) select an optimal treatment modality, and (4) document this process quickly and in a clear and precise manner. A predesigned SOAP form (subjective objective assessment plan) is often used to enhance the (1) rapid collection and systematic organization of important clinical data, (2) formulation of an assessment, and (3) selection of a treatment plan (Fig. 1-4).

Respiratory Assessment Immediately after the respiratory care practitioner systematically collects and documents the appropriate clinical data (clinical indicators), an

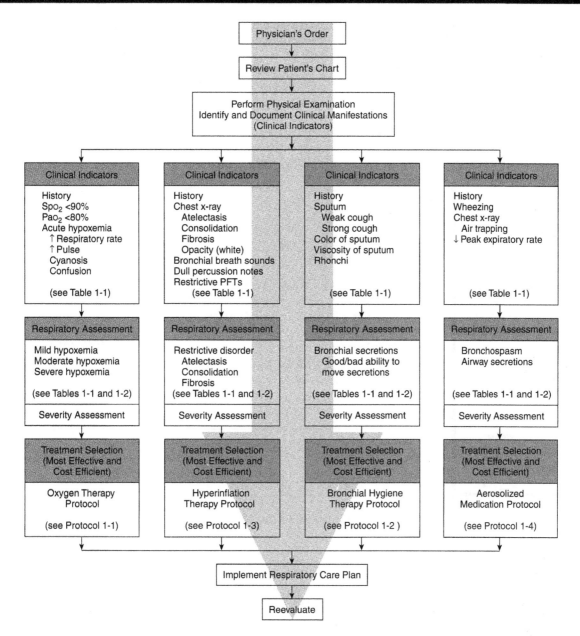

Fig. 1-2 Overview of the TDP program.

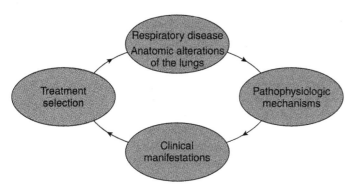

Fig. 1-3 Foundations for a strong TDP program. Overview of the knowledge base essential for assessment of respiratory diseases.

Subjective →	Objective →	Assessment →	Plan →
	Vital signs: RR __28__ HR __11__ BP __170/110__		Present Plan
"It feels like someone is standing on my chest."	Temp. __—__ On antipyretic agent? ☐ Yes ☐ No		
	Chest assessment:		
	Insp. *Use of accessory muscles of inspiration and pursed-lip breathing*		*None*
"I just can't seem to take a deep breath."			
	Palp. __—__		
	Perc. *Hyperresonant*		
Anterior	Ausc. *Expiratory wheezing and rhonchi bilaterally*	*Bronchospasm* *Large airway secretions*	**Plan Modifications**
R L	Radiography *Severely depressed diaphragm*	*Air trapping*	*Bronchodilator Tx per protocol*
Posterior	Bedside spir.: PEFR ā __165__ p̄ __—__ Tx		
	SVC____ FVC____ NIF____		
L R	Cough: ☐ Strong ☒ Weak	*Poor ability to mobilize thick secretions*	*CPT & PD per protocol*
Pt. name __—__	Sputum production: ☒ Yes ☐ No		
	Sputum char. *Large amt. thick/white secretions*		*Mucolytics per protocol*
Age __26__	Male __X__	Female			
Date __—__	Time¹ __—__	ABG: pH __7.27__ PaCO₂ __62__ HCO₃⁻ __25__	*Acute ventilatory failure with severe hypoxemia*	*Mechanical ventilation per protocol*
	PaO₂ __49__ SaO₂ __—__ SpO₂ __—__		
Admitting diagnosis *Asthma*	Neg. O₂ transport factors __—__		
Therapist __—__	Other: __—__		
Hospital __—__			*ABG in 30 minutes & reassess*

Respiratory Assessment Flow Chart

Fig. 1-4 Predesigned SOAP form.

assessment of the data must be formulated. For the most part, the assessment is primarily directed at the anatomic alterations of the lungs that are causing the clinical indicators (e.g., bronchospasm) and the severity of the clinical indicators.

Clinical Indicators and their Relationship to the Anatomic Alterations of the Lungs   The identification of specific anatomic alterations of the lungs that activate specific pathophysiologic mechanisms, which in turn lead to specific (and predictable) clinical manifestations, is an important part of the assessment process (see Fig. 1-3). Table 1-1 presents clinical indicators and assessments commonly made by the respiratory care practitioner.

An appropriate anatomic alteration of the lungs assessment for the clinical indicator of *wheezing* might be *bronchospasm*. If the practitioner assesses the cause of the wheezing correctly (in this example, bronchospasm), the appropriate treatment selection would be a bronchodilator agent from the *Aerosolized Medication Protocol.* However, if the cause of the wheezing was correctly assessed to be excessive airway secretions, the appropriate treatment plan would entail a specific treatment modality under the *Bronchial Hygiene Therapy Protocol,* including cough and deep breathing or chest physical therapy.

Table 1-1

Assessments and Treatment Selections Commonly Made by the Respiratory Care Practitioner

Objective Clinical Data	Assessments	Plan
Vital Signs		
↑breathing rate, ↑blood pressure, ↑pulse	Respiratory distress	Treat underlying cause
Airways		
Wheezing	Bronchospasm	Bronchodilator treatment
Inspiratory stridor	Laryngeal edema	Cool mist
Rhonchi	Secretions in large airways	Bronchial hygiene treatment
Crackles	Secretions in distal airways	Treat underlying cause—e.g., congestive heart failure (CHF)
		Hyperinflation treatment
Cough		
Strong cough	Good ability to mobilize secretions	None
Weak cough	Poor ability to mobilize secretions	Bronchial hygiene treatment
Secretions		
Amount: >30 ml/24 hrs	Excessive bronchial secretions	Bronchial hygiene treatment
White and translucent sputum	Normal sputum	None
Yellow or opaque sputum	Acute airway infection	Treat underlying cause
Green sputum	Old, retained secretions and infections	Bronchial hygiene treatment
Brown sputum	Old blood	Bronchial hygiene treatment
Red sputum	Fresh blood	Notify physician
Frothy secretions	Pulmonary edema	Treat underlying cause—e.g., CHF
		Hyperinflation treatment
Alveoli		
Bronchial breath sounds	Atelectasis	
Dull percussion note	Infiltrates	Hyperinflation treatment, oxygen treatment
Opacity on chest x-ray	Fibrosis	
Restrictive pulmonary function test values	Consolidation	No specific, effective respiratory care treatment
Depressed diaphragm on x-ray	Air trapping and hyperinflation	Treat underlying cause
Pleural Space		
Hyperresonant percussion note	Pneumothorax	Evacuate air* and hyperinflation treatment
Dull percussion note	Pleural effusion	Evacuate fluid* and hyperinflation treatment
Thorax		
Paradoxical movement of the chest wall	Flail chest	Mechanical ventilation*
Barrel chest	Air trapping (hyperinflation)	Treat underlying cause—e.g., asthma
Posterior and lateral curvature of spine	Kyphoscoliosis	Bronchial hygiene treatment
Arterial Blood Gases— Ventilatory		
pH ↑, $PaCO_2$↓, HCO_3^-↓	Acute alveolar hyperventilation	Treat underlying cause
pH N, $PaCO_2$↓, HCO_3^-↓↓	Chronic alveolar hyperventilation	Generally none
pH ↓, $PaCO_2$↑, HCO_3^-↑	Acute ventilatory failure	Mechanical ventilation*
pH N, $PaCO_2$↑, HCO_3^-↑↑	Chronic ventilatory failure	Low-flow oxygen, bronchial hygiene

*These procedures should be performed only as ordered by the physician.

Continued

Table 1-1 TABLE

Assessments and Treatment Selections Commonly Made by the Respiratory Care Practitioner—cont'd

Objective Clinical Data	Assessments	Plan
Sudden Ventilatory Changes on Chronic Ventilatory Failure (CVF)		
pH ↑, $PaCO_2$↑, HCO_3^- ↑↑, PaO_2↓	Acute alveolar hyperventilation on CVF	Treat underlying cause
pH ↓, $PaCO_2$↑↑, HCO_3^- ↑, PaO_2↓	Acute ventilatory failure on CVF	Mechanical ventilation*
Metabolic		
pH ↑, $PaCO_2$N or ↑, HCO_3^-↑, PaO_2N	Metabolic alkalosis	Give potassium*—Hypokalemia
		Give chloride*—Hypochloremia
pH ↓, $PaCO_2$N or ↓, HCO_3^-↓, PaO_2↓	Metabolic acidosis	Give oxygen—Lactic acidosis
pH ↓, $PaCO_2$N or ↓, HCO_3^-↓, PaO_2N	Metabolic acidosis	Give insulin*—Ketoacidosis
pH ↓, $PaCO_2$N or ↓, HCO_3^-↓, PaO_2N	Metabolic acidosis	Renal therapy*
Indication for Mechanical Ventilation		
pH ↑, $PaCO_2$↓, HCO_3^-↓, PaO_2↓	Impending ventilatory failure	
pH ↓, $PaCO_2$↑, HCO_3^-↑, PaO↓	Ventilatory failure	Mechanical ventilation*
pH ↓, $PaCO_2$↑, HCO_3^-↑, PaO_2↓	Apnea	
Oxygenation Status		
PaO_2 <80 mm Hg	Mild hypoxemia	
PaO_2 <60 mm Hg	Moderate hypoxemia	Oxygen treatment and treat underlying cause
PaO_2 <40 mm Hg	Severe hypoxemia	
Oxygen Transport Status		
↓ PaO_2, anemia, ↓ cardiac output	Inadequate oxygen transport	Oxygen treatment and treat underlying cause

These procedures should be performed only as ordered by the physician.

Severity Assessment The appropriate regulation of the frequency at which a respiratory therapy modality is to be administered is just as important as the selection of a respiratory therapy treatment. Often the frequency of treatment needs to be up-regulated or down-regulated on a shift-by-shift, hour-to-hour, minute-to-minute, or even (in life-threatening situations) second-to-second basis. Such frequency changes must be made in response to a basic systematic severity assessment. In a good TDP program, the well-seasoned respiratory care practitioner–the practitioner with extensive *clinical experience* and good *clinical judgment*–routinely and systematically documents many severity assessments throughout each working day.

For the new practitioner, however, a predesigned Severity Assessment Rating Form may be used to enhance this important part of the assessment process. One excellent, semiquantitative method of accomplishing this is illustrated in Table 1-2. For example, consider the Severity Assessment for the case on p. 11.

Fig. 1-5 illustrates the way a strong knowledge base of the major respiratory disorders and the assessment process and a good TDP program correlate.

Table 1-2

Respiratory Care Protocol Severity Assessment

Item	0 Points	1 Point	2 Points	3 Points	4 Points	Total
Respiratory history	Negative for smoking or history not available	Smoking history < pack a day	Smoking history > pack a day	Pulmonary disease	Severe or exacerbation	
Surgical history	None	General	Lower abdominal	Thoracic or upper abdominal	Thoracic with lung disease	
Level of consciousness	Alert, oriented, co-operative	Disoriented, follows commands	Obtunded, uncooperative	Obtunded	Comatose	
Level of activity	Ambulatory	Ambulatory with assistance	Nonambulatory	Paraplegic	Quadriplegic	
Respiratory pattern	Normal rate 8-20	Respiratory rate 20-25	Patient complains of dyspnea	Dyspnea, use of accessory muscles, prolonged expiration	Severe dyspnea, use of accessory muscles, respiratory rate >25, and/or shallow	
Breath sounds	Clear	Bilateral crackles	Bilateral crackles and rhonchi	Bilateral wheezing, crackles, and rhonchi	Absent and/or diminished bilateral and/or severe wheezing, crackles, or rhonchi	

Continued

Table 1-2

Respiratory Care Protocol Severity Assessment—cont'd

Item	0 Points	1 Point	2 Points	3 Points	4 Points	Total
Cough	Strong, spontaneous, nonproductive	Excessive bronchial secretions and strong cough	Excessive bronchial secretions but weak cough	Thick bronchial secretions and weak cough	Thick bronchial secretions but no cough	
Chest x-ray	Clear	One lobe: infiltrates, atelectasis, consolidation, or pleural effusion	Same lung, two lobes: infiltrates, atelectasis, consolidation, or pleural effusion	One lobe in both lungs: infiltrates, atelectasis, consolidation, or pleural effusion	Both lungs, more than one lobe: infiltrates, atelectasis, consolidation, or pleural effusion	
Arterial blood gases and/or oxygen saturation measured by pulse oximetry (SpO_2)	Normal	Normal pH and $PaCO_2$, but PaO_2 60-80 and/or SpO_2 91-96	Normal pH and $PaCO_2$, but PaO_2 40-60 and/or SpO_2 85-90	Acute respiratory alkalosis, PaO_2 <40 and/or SpO_2 80-84	Acute respiratory failure, PaO_2 <80 and/or SpO_2 <80	

Severity Index

Total Score	Severity Assessment	Treatment Frequency
1-5	Unremarkable	As needed
6-15	Mild	Two or three times a day
16-25	Moderate	Four times a day or as needed
Greater than 26	Severe	Two to four times a day and as needed Alert attending physician

Severity Assessment Case Example

A 67-year-old man arrived in the emergency room in respiratory distress. The patient was well known to the TDP team; he had been diagnosed with chronic bronchitis several years before this admission (3 points). The patient had no recent surgery history, and he was ambulatory, alert, and cooperative (0 points). He complained of dyspnea and was using his accessory muscles of inspiration (3 points). Auscultation revealed bilateral rhonchi over both lung fields (3 points). His cough was weak and productive of thick, grey secretions (3 points). A chest x-ray revealed pneumonia (consolidation) in the left lower lung lobe (3 points). On room air his arterial blood gas values were as follows: pH 7.52, $PaCO_2$ 54, HCO_3^- 41, and PaO_2 52—acute alveolar hyperventilation on chronic ventilatory failure (3 points).

Using the Severity Assessment Form shown in table 1-2, the following treatment selection and administration frequency would be appropriate:

Severity Assessment

Total score: 17
Treatment selection: Chest physical therapy
Frequency of administration: Four times a day and as needed

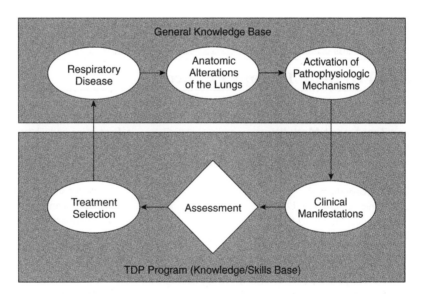

Fig. 1-5 The way knowledge, assessment, and a TDP program interface.

TREATMENT PROTOCOLS COMMONLY SELECTED BY THE RESPIRATORY PRACTITIONER

The treatment portion of a TDP is based on selection of treatment procedures that work to correct or offset the anatomic alterations and pathophysiologic mechanisms caused by the respiratory disorder and are most cost effective. However, the treatment portion (e.g., Bronchial Hygiene Therapy Protocol) is only part of the TDP. Before a specific treatment modality can be started, specific clinical indicators (objective data) must first be identified and documented to justify the therapy given to the patient (see Fig. 1-5).

Top Four Treatment Protocol Categories

The essential foundation of a successful TDP program is based on four treatment protocol categories: the *Oxygen Therapy Protocol* (Protocol 1-1), *Bronchial Hygiene Therapy Protocol* (Protocol 1-2), *Hyperinflation Therapy Protocol* (Protocol 1-3), and *Aerosolized Medication Protocol* (Protocol 1-4).

Each treatment protocol has several different treatment modalities (officially approved by the medical staff and hospital administration). In essence, the treat-

---

Protocol **1-1**

Oxygen Therapy Protocol

Objective
To treat hypoxemia, decrease the work of breathing, and decrease myocardial work

Common Treatment Modalities
- Nasal cannula
- Oxygen mask
- Venturi mask
- Partial rebreathing mask
- Nonrebreathing mask
- Patient education (if discharge planning or home care is in process)

Protocol **1-2**

Bronchial Hygiene Therapy Protocol

Objective
To enhance mobilization of bronchial secretions

Common Treatment Modalities
- Increased bronchial hydration
    Increased fluid intake (6 to 10 glasses of water a day)
    Bland aerosol therapy
    Ultrasonic nebulization (USN)
- Cough and deep breathing (C&DB)
    Techniques used to enhance C&DB
      Incentive spirometry (IS)
      Intermittent positive pressure breathing (IPPB)
      Positive expiratory pressure (PEP) therapy
      Flutter valve
- Chest physical therapy (CPT)
- Postural drainage (PD)
- Percussion and vibration with postural drainage
- Suctioning
- Mucolytic therapy (see Protocol 1-4)
    Acetylcysteine (Mucomyst)—often in combination with a bronchodilator
    Recombinant human deoxyribonuclease I (DNase, Pulmozyme)
    Sodium bicarbonate (2% solution)
    Assistance to physician in bronchoscopy
- Patient education (if discharge planning or home care is in process)

An example of a typical algorithm for the Bronchial Hygiene Therapy Protocol is presented in Fig. 1-6.

Protocol **1-3**

Hyperinflation Therapy Protocol

Objective
To prevent or treat alveolar consolidation and atelectasis

Common Treatment Modalities
- Cough and deep breathing (C&DB)
- Incentive spirometry (IS)
- Intermittent positive pressure breathing (IPPB)
- Continuous positive airway pressure (CPAP)
- Positive end-expiratory pressure (PEEP)
- Patient education (if discharge planning or home care is in process)

ment modalities listed below each protocol category serve as a treatment selection menu. When the patient demonstrates the clinical indicators for any of the TDPs, the respiratory therapist working in the program is expected to select and administer the most appropriate and cost-effective treatment modalities to the patient.

The treatment selection and frequency with which the therapy is administered is based on (1) the severity of the clinical manifestations demonstrated by the patient, (2) the patient's ability to perform or tolerate the therapy, and (3) the patient's response to the therapy. For example, the Hyperinflation Therapy Protocol is a general treatment protocol category designed to prevent or correct atelectasis after thoracic surgery. However, if the patient is unconscious or unable to follow directions, a continuous positive airway pressure (CPAP) mask is a more appropriate treatment selection (under the Hyperinflation Therapy Protocol) than, say, incentive spirometry—even though both are designed to treat or prevent atelectasis. Fig. 1-6 provides an example of a typical treatment protocol algorithm for the Bronchial Hygiene Therapy Protocol.

Mechanical Ventilation Protocol—the Fifth Protocol

Even when the patient is transferred to the intensive care unit and placed on a mechanical ventilator, the respiratory care practitioner must usually still administer one or more of the four respiratory therapy treatment protocols (e.g., Hyperinflation

---

Protocol **1-4**

Aerosolized Medication Protocol

Bronchodilator
Objective
Sympathomimetics and parasympatholytics—to offset bronchial smooth muscle constriction
Common Treatment Modalities
   Sympathomimetics
   • Albuterol (Ventolin, Proventil)
   • Metaproterenol (Alupent, Metaprel)
   • Terbutaline (Brethine, Brethaire)
   • Pirbuterol (Maxair)
   • Salmeterol (Serevent)
   Parasympatholytics (anticholinergic)
   • Atropine sulfate (Dey-Dose Atropine Sulfate)
   • Ipratropium bromide (Atrovent)
Mucolytic Agents
Objective
Mucolytic agents—to enhance the mobilization and thinning of bronchial secretions
Common Treatment Modalities
   • Acetylcysteine (Mucomyst)
   • Recombinant human deoxyribonuclease (DNase, Pulmozyme)
   • Sodium bicarbonate (2% solution)

Antiinflammatory Agents
Objective
Aerosolized corticosteroids—to suppress bronchial inflammation and edema; also used for their ability to enhance the responsiveness of B_2 receptor sites to sympathomimetic agents
Common Treatment Modalities
   • Dexamethasone (Decadron Respihaler)
   • Beclomethasone (Vanceril, Beclovent)
   • Triamcinolone (Azmacort)
   • Flunisolide (AeroBid)
Antibiotic Agents
Objective
Antibiotics—to treat infectious respiratory diseases
Common Treatment Modalities
   • Gentamicin (commonly used in treatment of cystic fibrosis)
   • Tobramycin (commonly used in treatment of cystic fibrosis)
   • Pentamidine (*Pneumocystis carinii* pneumonia)
   • Ribavirin (respiratory syncytial virus)
   • Patient education (if discharge planning or home care is in process)

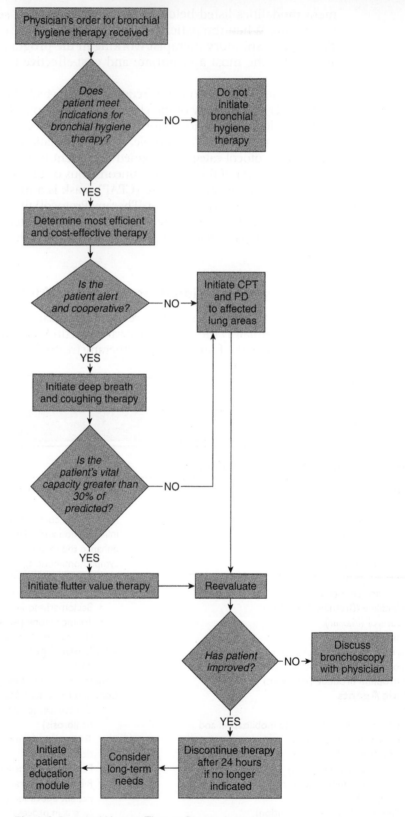

Fig. 1-6 Bronchial Hygiene Therapy Protocol algorithm.

Protocol **1-5**   PROTOCOL

Mechanical Ventilation Protocol

Objective
To provide and support alveolar gas exchange and eventually return the patient to spontaneous breathing

Common Treatment Modalities
- Airway establishment (intubation) and management
- Cuff management
- Ventilatory management
  - Respiratory rate (frequency), tidal volume
  - Oxygen concentration (FiO_2) (see Table 1-1)

- Ventilator system pressure (peak, mean, positive end-expiratory pressure [PEEP], continuous positive airway pressure [CPAP])
- Ventilator mode (intermittent mechanical ventilation [IMV], synchronized intermittent mechanical ventilation [SIMV], pressure support)
- Weaning strategies
- Patient education (if discharge planning or home care is in process)

Therapy Protocol via CPAP or positive end-expiratory pressure [PEEP], or an in-line aerosolized medication, such as a bronchodilator). For the purpose of this workbook, the authors have chosen to refer to Mechanical Ventilation Protocol as the *Fifth Protocol* (Protocol 1-5). The high-technology, high-risk, high-visibility portion of respiratory care work is clearly embedded in ventilator management. Much of the success of the TDP movement has occurred because of the dramatic ways in which standardized, data-driven algorithms have improved patient outcomes. Most dramatic are hastened ventilator weaning times, reduction of nosocomial infections, and reduced complication rates of mechanical ventilation (e.g., barotrauma).

To summarize the essential components of the assessment process, Fig. 1-7 provides an assessment form with common examples for each category—that is, clinical indicators, respiratory assessments, and treatment plans. The examples shown in Fig. 1-7 can easily be transferred to the SOAP format. The SOAP format used in the assessment of respiratory diseases is discussed in more detail in Chapter 10 of *Clinical Manifestations and Assessment of Respiratory Disease*.

COMMON RESPIRATORY DISORDERS SEEN IN A TDP PROGRAM

Although the respiratory care practitioner may treat one or two cases of every respiratory disorder presented in this book, most of the professional's career will be spent caring for only a few of them. As much as 80% of the respiratory practitioner's work is concerned with intelligent assessment and treatment selection for a short list of respiratory illnesses (Table 1-3).

Common Anatomic Alterations of the Lungs

Common anatomic alterations of the lungs treated by the respiratory care practitioner can be derived by noting of the respiratory disorders presented in Table 1-3. The major anatomic alterations include (1) *atelectasis* (e.g., after upper abdominal or thoracic surgery), (2) *consolidation* (e.g., pneumonia), (3) *increased alveolar-capillary membrane* (e.g., adult respiratory distress syndrome [ARDS], pulmonary edema), (4) *bronchospasm* (e.g., asthma), (5) *bronchial secretions* (e.g., bronchitis, asthma, pulmonary edema), and (6) *distal airway and alveolar weakening* (e.g., emphysema).

| Patient Identification Box | Date:_____ | Admitting Diagnosis:_____ |
| | Time:_____ | Attending Physician:_____ |

Clinical Indicators (see Table 1-1)			
Oxygen Therapy	Bronchial Hygiene Therapy	Hyperinflation Therapy	Aerosolized Medication Bronchodilator Agent

Examples:
 	
☐ History
☐ Spo_2 <80%
☐ Pao_2 <80%
☐ Acute hypoxemia
  ☐ ↑ Respiratory rate
  ☐ ↑ Pulse
  ☐ Cyanosis
  ☐ Confusion
  ☐ Other
	Examples:
	
	☐ History
	☐ Sputum
	  ☐ Weak cough
	  ☐ Color of sputum
	  ☐ Viscosity of sputum
	  ☐ Rhonchi
		Examples:
		
		☐ History
		☐ Chest x-ray
		  ☐ Atelectasis
		  ☐ Consolidation
		  ☐ Fibrosis
		  ☐ Opacity (white)
		☐ Bronchial breath sounds
		☐ Restrictive PFT values
			Examples:
			
			☐ History
			☐ Wheezing
			☐ Chest x-ray
			  ☐ Air trapping
			☐ Obstructive PFT values

Respiratory Assessments (see Tables 1-1 and 1-2)			
Oxygen Therapy	Bronchial Hygiene Therapy	Hyperinflation Therapy	Aerosolized Medication
Examples: ☐ Mild hypoxemia ☐ Moderate hypoxemia ☐ Severe hypoxemia Severity Score:_____	Examples: ☐ Excessive sputum production ☐ Thick secretions ☐ Weak cough Severity Score:_____	Examples: ☐ Atelectasis ☐ Consolidation ☐ Weak diaphragm Severity Score:_____	Examples: ☐ Bronchospasm ☐ Thick secretions ☐ Bronchial edema Severity Score:_____

Treatment Plans			
Oxygen Therapy (see Protocol 1-1)	Bronchial Hygiene Therapy (see Protocol 1-2)	Hyperinflation Therapy (see Protocol 1-3)	Aerosolized Medication (see Protocol 1-4)
Examples: ☐ Nasal cannula ☐ Oxygen mask ☐ 28% Venturi mask Frequency:_____	Examples: ☐ Deep breath and cough ☐ Chest physical therapy ☐ Postural drainage Frequency:_____	Examples: ☐ Incentive spirometry ☐ CPAP ☐ PEEP Frequency:_____	Examples: ☐ Ventolin ☐ Vanceril ☐ Acetylcysteine Frequency:_____

| Reevaluation Date:_____ | Therapist Signature:_____ |

Fig. 1-7 Respiratory care protocol program assessment form.

Table 1-3

Common Respiratory Disorders

Respiratory Disorder	DRG Number*
Chronic bronchitis, emphysema	88
Asthma	97
Acute pneumonia	79, 89, 90
Aspiration pneumonia	80
Atelectasis	101/102
Adult respiratory distress syndrome	99/102
Congestive heart failure/pulmonary edema	127
Respiratory failure	87
Respiratory failure with ventilatory support	475
Respiratory failure/tracheostomy/ventilatory support	483

*Respiratory disorders can be identified by their respective diagnosis-related group (DRG). DRG is an identification system used to categorize and document diseases, primarily for use in health care reimbursement (such as Medicaid and Medicare). Patients are routinely assigned a DRG based on their admitting diagnosis, and each DRG communicates information about patients. Because the use of DRGs is prevalent, respiratory care practitioners should recognize and understand the DRGs they will commonly encounter.

Box 1-1

Pathophysiologic Mechanisms Commonly Activated in Respiratory Disorders

- Decreased ventilation/perfusion ($\dot{V}/\dot{Q}$) ratio
- Alveolar diffusion block
- Decreased lung compliance
- Stimulation of oxygen receptors
- Deflation reflex
- Irritant reflex
- Pulmonary reflex
- Increased airway resistance
- Air trapping and alveolar hyperinflation

CLINICAL SCENARIOS ACTIVATED BY COMMON ANATOMIC ALTERATIONS OF THE LUNGS

Specific anatomic alterations of the lung (such as the ones listed previously) lead to the activation of specific and predictable pathophysiologic mechanisms. The more common pathophysiologic mechanisms are listed in Box 1-1. The pathophysiologic mechanisms, in turn, activate at specific and predictable clinical manifestations (see Fig. 1-3). *For the purposes of this workbook, the authors have chosen to refer to the interrelationship among the major anatomic alterations of the lung, the pathophysiologic mechanisms, and the clinical manifestations that result as* clinical scenarios. To enhance the reader's knowledge and understanding of commonly encountered respiratory disorders, clinical scenarios for the anatomic alterations presented in the following paragraphs are provided.*

*The Case Study Discussion Section at the end of each respiratory disease chapter often refers the reader back to these clinical scenarios—correlating various clinical manifestations to specific pathophysiologic mechanisms and anatomic alterations of the lungs.

Key to Abbreviations in Figs. 1-8 Through 1-13

ABG	= Arterial blood gas
ARDS	= Adult respiratory distress syndrome
CPAP	= Continuous positive airway pressure
CPT	= Chest physical therapy
Do_2	= Total oxygen delivery
ERV	= Expiratory reserve volume
FEF	= Forced expiratory flow, midexpiratory phase
FEV_1	= Forced expiratory volume in 1 second
FEVT	= Forced expiratory volume, timed
FRC	= Functional residual capacity
FVC	= Forced vital capacity
IC	= Inspiratory capacity
MVV	= Maximum voluntary ventilation
O_2ER	= Oxygen extraction ratio
PD	= Postural drainage
PEEP	= Positive end-expiratory pressure
PEFR	= Peak expiratory flow rate
PFT	= Pulmonary function test
$\dot{Q}s/\dot{Q}_T$	= Cardiac output shunted/total cardiac output
RV	= Residual volume
$S\bar{v}o_2$	= Mixed venous oxygen saturation
TLC	= Total lung capacity
VC	= Vital capacity
$\dot{V}/\dot{Q}$	= Ventilation/perfusion

Atelectasis

Fig. 1-8 shows the pathophysiologic mechanisms caused by atelectasis (such as that occurring after thoracic surgery), the clinical manifestations that result, and the treatment protocols used to offset them. The hypoxemia that results from atelectasis is caused by capillary shunting. This type of hypoxemia is refractory to oxygen therapy. Therefore the implementation of the Hyperinflation Therapy Protocol may be more beneficial in the treatment of hypoxemia than the Oxygen Therapy Protocol for the patient with atelectasis.

Alveolar Consolidation

Fig. 1-9 shows the pathophysiologic mechanisms caused by alveolar consolidation (e.g., pneumonia), the clinical manifestations that result, and the treatment protocols used to offset them. The hypoxemia that develops as a result of consolidation is caused by capillary shunting. This type of hypoxemia is refractory to oxygen therapy.

Depending on the severity of the alveolar consolidation, the Hyperinflation Therapy Protocol or the Oxygen Therapy Protocol may be beneficial. In general, however, there is no effective, specific respiratory care treatment modality for alveolar consolidation. With pneumonia the great temptation for the respiratory care practitioner is to do too much, such as instituting hyperinflation therapy, bronchodilator therapy, and bronchial hygiene therapy. Such treatment protocols generally are not indicated, especially during the early stages. Appropriate antibiotics (prescribed by the physician), bed rest, fluids, and supplementary oxygen are all that is usually

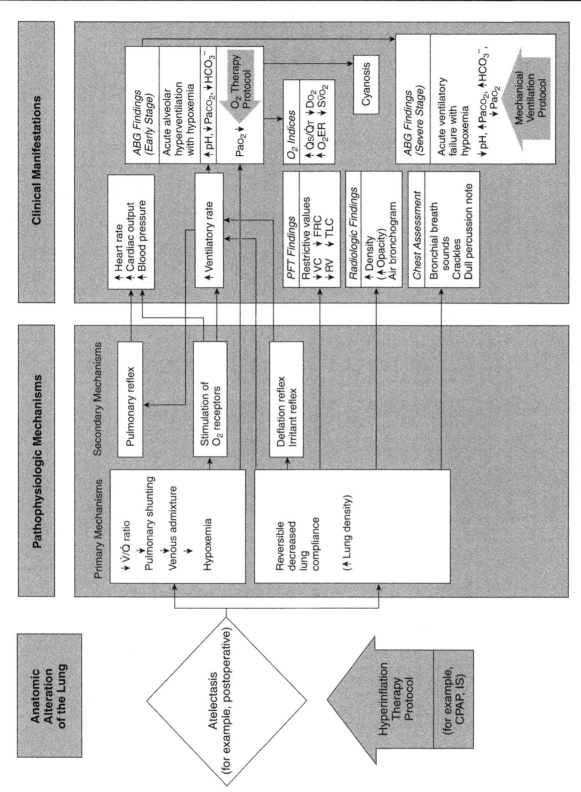

Fig. 1-8 Atelectasis clinical scenario.

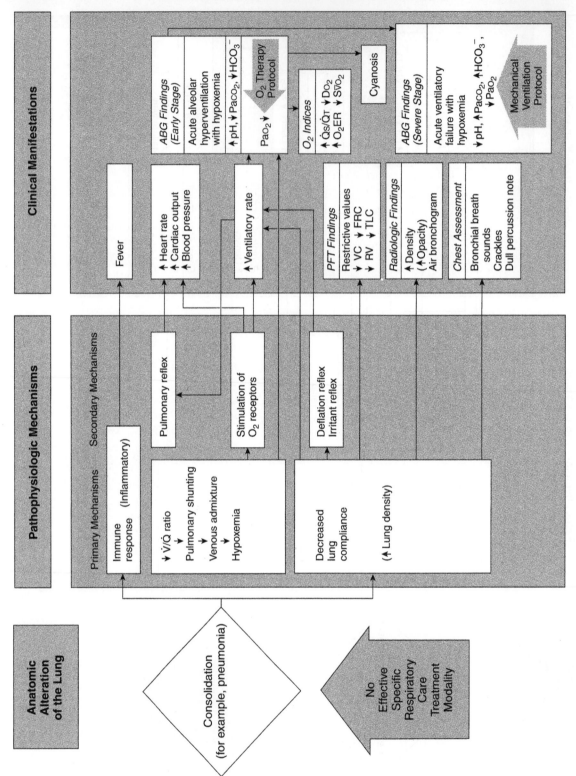

Fig. 1-9 Alveolar Consolidation clinical scenario.

needed. When pneumonia is in its resolution stage, however, there may be excessive secretions and atelectasis, accompanied by bronchoconstriction. At this time, other treatment modalities may be indicated.

Increased Alveolar-Capillary Membrane Thickness

Fig. 1-10 illustrates the major pathophysiologic mechanisms caused by increased alveolar-capillary membrane thickness (e.g., postoperative ARDS, asbestosis, chronic interstitial lung disease), the clinical manifestations that develop, and the treatment protocols used to offset them. The hypoxemia that develops as a result of an increased alveolar-capillary membrane thickness is caused by an alveolar diffusion block. This type of hypoxemia often responds favorably to oxygen therapy.

Bronchospasm

Fig. 1-11 shows the major pathophysiologic mechanisms activated by bronchospasm (e.g., asthma), the clinical manifestations that result, and the appropriate treatment protocols used to offset them. The Aerosolized Medication Therapy Protocol (Bronchodilator Therapy) is the primary treatment modality used to offset the anatomic alterations of bronchospasm (the original cause of the pathophysiologic chain of events). The *Oxygen Therapy Protocol* and *Mechanical Ventilation Protocol* are secondary treatment modalities used to offset the mild, moderate, or severe clinical manifestations associated with bronchospasm. In other words, when the patient responds favorably to the *Aerosolized Medication Therapy Protocol*, the need for the *Oxygen Therapy Protocol* may be minimal and the *Mechanical Ventilation Protocol* may not be necessary at all.

Excessive Bronchial Secretions

Fig. 1-12 illustrates the major pathophysiologic mechanisms caused by excessive bronchial secretions (e.g., chronic bronchitis, asthma), the clinical manifestations that result, and the appropriate treatment protocols used to correct them. When the patient demonstrates chronic ventilatory failure during the advanced stages of respiratory disorders associated with chronic excessive bronchial secretions (e.g., chronic bronchitis), caution must be taken not to over-oxygenate the patient.

Distal Airway and Alveolar Weakening

Fig. 1-13 illustrates the major pathophysiologic mechanisms caused by distal airway and alveolar weakening (e.g., emphysema), the clinical manifestations that result, and the appropriate treatment protocols used to offset them. Pulmonary rehabilitation and oxygen therapy may be all the practitioner can provide to treat disorders associated with distal airway and alveolar weakening. When the patient demonstrates chronic ventilatory failure during the advanced stages of the disorder, caution must be taken with the *Oxygen Therapy Protocol* not to over-oxygenate the patient.

When the respiratory therapy practitioner knows and understands the chain of events (clinical scenarios) that develop in response to common anatomic alterations of the lungs, an assessment and an appropriate treatment protocol can easily be determined. Fig. 1-14 provides a three-component overview model of a prototype airway to further enhance the reader's visualization of anatomic alterations of the lungs commonly associated with respiratory disorders and the treatment plans commonly used to offset them.

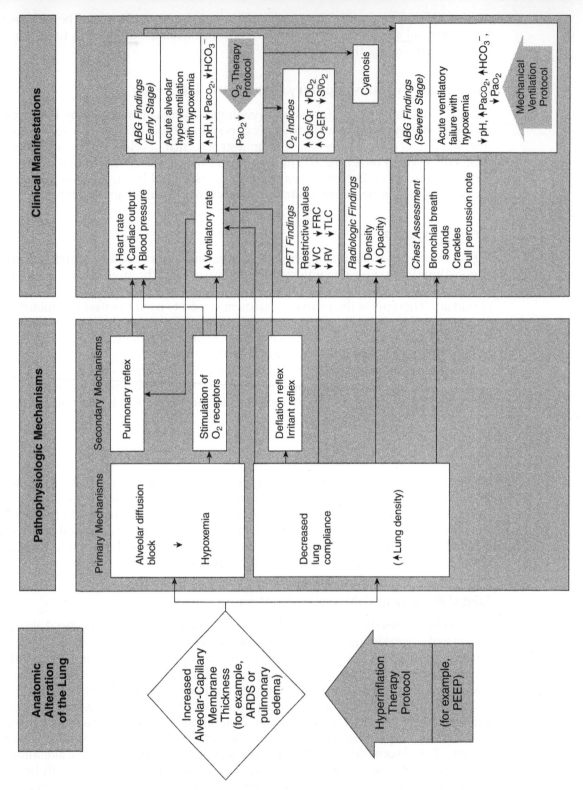

Fig. 1-10 Increased Alveolar-Capillary Membrane Thickness clinical scenario.

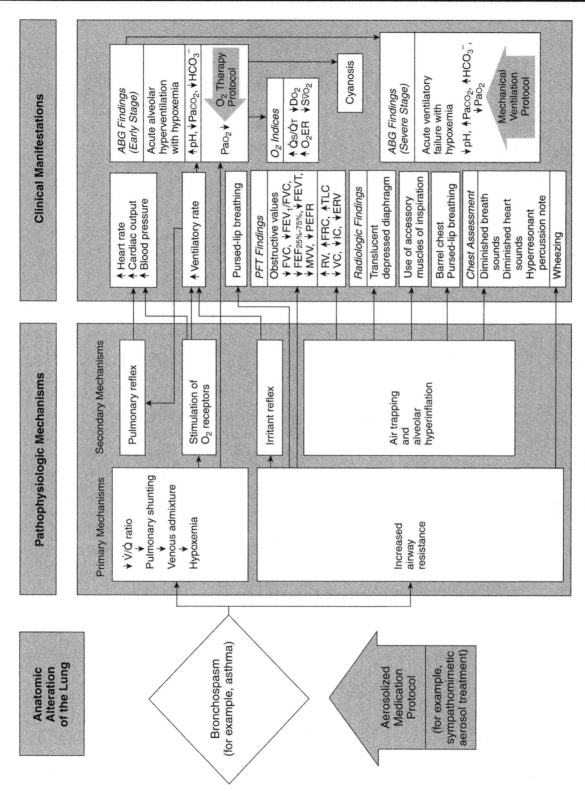

Fig. 1-11 Bronchospasm clinical scenario.

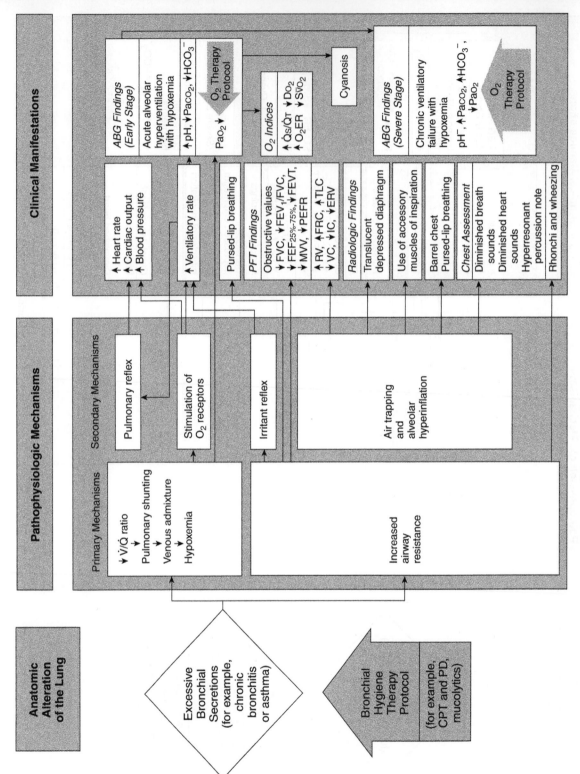

Fig. I-12 Excessive Bronchial Secretions clinical scenario.

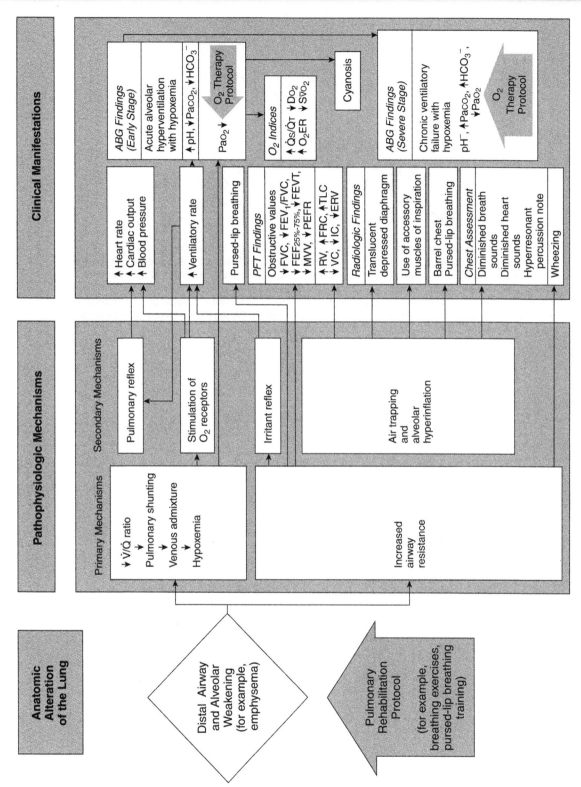

Fig. 1-13 Distal Airway and Alveolar Weakening clinical scenario.

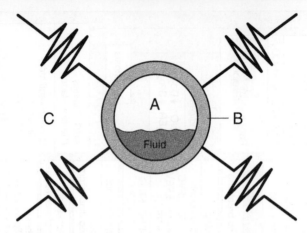

Fig. 1-14 A three-component model of a prototype airway. Therapy may be directed to any or all components. *A*, Airway lumen; *B*, airway wall; *C*, supporting structures. Therapy for *A* includes deep breathing and coughing, smoking cessation, suctioning, mucolytics, bland aerosols, systemic and parenteral hydration, and therapeutic bronchoscopy. Therapy for *B* includes bronchodilators, aerosolized antiinflammatory agents, aerosolized antibiotics, and aerosolized decongestants. Therapy for *C* includes pursed-lip breathing exercises and removal of external factors compressing the airway (bullae, pleural effusion, pneumothorax, tumor masses).

PART II

Obstructive Airway Diseases

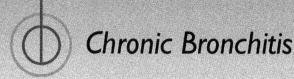

Chronic Bronchitis

ADMITTING HISTORY

A 68-year-old retired geologist arrived in the emergency room with his daughter. Well known to the respiratory care consult team, he has a 40-year history of smoking a pack of cigarettes a day, is widowed, lives alone, and has difficulty managing his daily activities. For the past week the man has experienced increased dyspnea and cough and has been unable to care for himself. On observation his personal hygiene appeared to have deteriorated. The man stated that he has been unable to get his breath or inhale deep enough to cough up secretions. He complained of mild nausea without abdominal pain or vomiting. His physician had given him an unknown oral antibiotic 3 days before this admission.

The man was diagnosed with severe chronic bronchitis approximately 6 years ago and had an acute myocardial infarction 2 years ago. His pulmonary function studies 1 year before this admission showed severe airway obstruction and air trapping. He has a history of high blood pressure, congestive heart failure, chronic dyspnea on exertion, and chronic cough, and he experienced two episodes of pneumonia within the last year. In recent months, according to a neighbor, he has become increasingly depressed.

According to his daughter, his physical activity is minimal. He generally spends most of his days watching television, smoking, and napping. All his children, none of whom live in the immediate area, have tried to coax him to move to a boardinghouse environment, but he has adamantly refused. During his last admission the advantages of pulmonary rehabilitation were discussed with him. The patient said that he had no need for pulmonary education, nor for the services of other agencies or organizations to check up on him in his home.

PHYSICAL EXAMINATION (TIME: 1730)

Inspection revealed a barrel chest, clubbing of his fingers and toes, cyanotic skin, and pitting edema (2+) around his ankles. His breathing was labored; he was pursed-lip breathing, using his accessory muscles of respiration, and he appeared weak. He had a frequent, weak cough productive of large amounts of thick, yellow sputum.

Vital signs were as follows: blood pressure 190/115, heart rate 125 bpm, respiratory rate 30/min, and oral temperature 37° C (98.6° F). Tactile fremitus was present over both lung fields, and hyperresonant percussion notes were produced both anteriorly and posteriorly. Bilateral rhonchi were auscultated. His abdomen was soft and not tender. Bowel sounds were active.

On room air his arterial blood gas values (ABGs) were as follows: pH 7.53, $Paco_2$ 56 mm Hg, HCO_3^- 33 mmol/L, and Pao_2 43 mm Hg. Review of his chart showed that on his last hospital discharge his baseline ABGs on 2 L/min oxygen were as follows: pH 7.39, $Paco_2$ 85 mm Hg, HCO_3^- 38 mmol/L, and Pao_2 64 mm Hg. His carboxyhemoglobin level was 6%. His chest x-ray on this admission showed severe hyperinflation with depressed hemidiaphragms. No acute infiltrates were apparent. His heart size was normal (Fig. 2-1). His complete blood count values were all normal except for a hematocrit of 58%. The attending physician ordered a respiratory care consult. The following order was written in the patient's chart: "All efforts should be made to keep the patient off the ventilator."

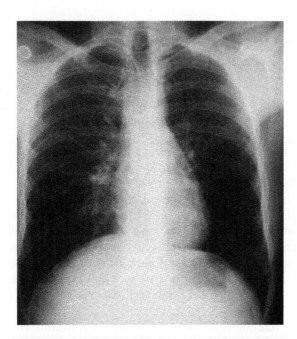

Fig. 2-1 Chest x-ray of a 68-year-old man with chronic bronchitis.

Response 1

Based on the previous information, write your SOAP in the following space:

S _____

_____

O _____

_____

Response 1 – cont'd

A

P

EARLY MORNING, NEXT DAY (TIME: 0230)

The respiratory care practitioner on duty was called by the floor nurse to evaluate the patient. The nurse reported that the patient had said that he was having a bad period. The nurse further thought that the patient appeared restless and short of breath and was coughing excessively.

On inspection the patient could be seen using his accessory muscles of respiration. He demonstrated pursed-lip breathing. In addition, he demonstrated a weak, productive cough and expectorated large amounts of thick, yellow secretions. The patient's vital signs were as follows: blood pressure 185/135, heart rate 130 bpm, respiratory rate 28/min, and oral temperature 37° C (98.6° F). Bilateral rhonchi were auscultated over the lung bases. His ABGs were as follows: pH 7.55, $PaCO_2$ 53 mm Hg, HCO_3^- 32 mmol/L, PaO_2 41 mm Hg. His hemoglobin oxygen saturation measured by pulse oximetry (SpO_2) was 83%.

Response 2

Based on the previous information, write your SOAP in the following space.

S _____

_____

O _____

_____

_____

_____

_____

_____

_____

A _____

_____

_____

_____

_____

_____

_____

_____

Response 2–cont'd

P _____

_____

_____

_____

_____

_____

LATE AFTERNOON, SAME DAY (TIME: 1415)

Although the patient had been resting comfortably for several hours, he suddenly became short of breath and difficult to arouse directly before a scheduled bronchial hygiene treatment. The respiratory therapist on duty noted that the patient said that he was "doing worse again." He was sitting up in bed and using his accessory muscles of respiration and pursed-lip breathing. His breathing was rapid and shallow. His cough continued to be weak. No sputum production was noted at this time. Expiration was prolonged.

His vital signs were as follows: blood pressure 150/95, heart rate 140 bpm, respiratory rate 25/min, and temperature 37° C (98.6° F). He had bilateral wheezes and rhonchi. A recent chest x-ray was unavailable. His ABGs were as follows: pH 7.28, $Paco_2$ 105 mm Hg, HCO_3^- 41 mmol/L, and Pao_2 44 mm Hg. His carboxyhemoglobin level was 2.5%. A toxic drug blood screen was negative.

Response 3

Based on the previous information, write your SOAP in the following space.

S _____

_____

O _____

_____

_____

Continued

Response 3—cont'd

_____

_____

_____

_____

_____

_____

A _____

_____

_____

_____

_____

_____

_____

_____

P _____

_____

_____

_____

_____

_____

_____

KEY POINT QUESTIONS

For Chronic Bronchitis (DRG* 88)

1. Basic Concept Formation
   a. What are the most common causes of chronic bronchitis?
   b. Are the *clinical manifestations* of cough and sputum production characteristic of this disorder? If so, why?
   c. How are secretions normally *cleared* from the airway?
   d. Are these mechanisms impaired in patients with chronic bronchitis?
   e. Does *smoking cessation* improve the symptoms of chronic bronchitis?
2. Database Formation
   a. What is your *vision* of the pathologic process of chronic bronchitis?
   b. Which *pathophysiologic mechanisms* are activated as a result of the typical anatomic alterations?
   c. Which portion(s) of the *airway model* (see Fig. 1-14) is/are abnormal in cases of chronic bronchitis?
   d. What are the *extrapulmonary signs and symptoms* of severe cases of chronic bronchitis?
   e. What should be the *goals of therapy* for such patients?
   f. Which *standard therapist-driven protocols* would achieve these goals?
   g. What are the expected *outcomes,* possible *adverse effects,* and *monitors* of the beneficial and adverse effects of the therapies you have selected?
3. Assessment
   a. Did the patient in this case study initially or subsequently demonstrate any evidence of the *clinical manifestations* of chronic bronchitis? What were they?
   b. Did the patient in this case study initially demonstrate any evidence of the *pathophysiologic alterations* associated with chronic bronchitis? What did this evidence include?
   c. Which *specific clinical manifestations* of chronic bronchitis did this patient initially demonstrate that helped you determine the *severity* of his condition?
4. Application
   a. Oxygen therapy (was/was not) indicated because _____ .
   b. Monitoring (was/was not) indicated because _____ .
   c. Aerosolized medication therapy (was/was not) indicated because _____ .
   d. Bronchial hygiene therapy (was/was not) indicated because _____ .
   e. Postural drainage (PD) and percussion (were/were not) indicated because _____ .
   f. Pulmonary rehabilitation (should/should not) be used in the comprehensive care of this patient because _____ .
5. Evaluation
   a. What are the expected outcomes of each aspect of therapy you have selected?
   b. How should you *monitor* patient response?
   c. What are the upper limits on the *intensity* and *frequency* of the administration of each therapeutic modality?
   d. What are the *advantages* and *disadvantages* of each treatment modality?
   e. What do you do if the patient improves?
   f. What do you do if he does not improve?

---

*DRG, *Diagnosis-related group.*

Continued

KEY POINT QUESTIONS—cont'd

6. Boundary Awareness
   a. How would you know if *this* patient's condition does not improve or worsens?
   b. When should you ask a supervisor for help?
   c. When should you call the patient's physician?
   d. How would you recognize actual or impending ventilatory failure in this patient?
   e. What adverse effects are possible with the treatments you have selected?

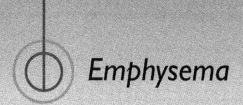

Emphysema

3

ADMITTING HISTORY

A 62-year-old man has a history of cough and shortness of breath, coupled with multiple hospitalizations. He was admitted because of severe, worsening dyspnea. He lived and worked in Pittsburgh, Pennsylvania, for 35 years as a foundry worker in a steel manufacturing plant. His wife died 10 years earlier. After his wife's death, he lived alone for 9 years and managed his daily activities with progressive difficulty.

Approximately 2 years before this admission he was forced to retire early because of declining health. His doctor told him that he had chronic emphysema. For the past year he has been living with his brother's family in Chicago. During the interview the patient's brother indicated that the man might "have the flu again." He has a 35 pack-year history of smoking unfiltered cigarettes, but he stopped smoking at the time of his forced retirement.

His last hospitalization was 9 weeks before this admission. At that time he was hospitalized for 2 days for cough, muscle aches and pains, fever, and respiratory distress. He underwent a complete pulmonary function study and received bronchial hygiene therapy, oxygen therapy, and instruction in at-home breathing exercises.

Also at this time, hospital personnel noted that the patient's expiratory flow rate measurements had declined significantly since his pulmonary function tests (PFTs) a year earlier. In fact, his forced expiratory volume in 1 second (FEV_1) had declined from 70% of predicted to 45% of predicted in the past year. At discharge 9 weeks before this admission and on 1.5 L/min oxygen by nasal cannula, the patient's arterial blood gas values (ABGs) were as follows: pH 7.37, $PaCO_2$ 67 mm Hg, HCO_3^- 36 mmol/L, and PaO_2 63 mm Hg. He had received an influenza vaccine 6 months earlier and a pneumococcal vaccine 2 years earlier.

At the time of discharge 9 weeks earlier he was pursed-lip breathing and using his accessory muscles of inspiration at rest. He demonstrated no spontaneous cough or sputum production. His bronchodilator therapy was discontinued 1 year ago because it had been found to be "ineffective" during his PFT. He was strongly encouraged to perform his pulmonary rehabilitation exercises daily. A weekly exercise flow chart was provided for him at discharge by the respiratory care department.

PHYSICAL EXAMINATION

In the emergency room the patient was febrile, cyanotic, and in obvious respiratory distress. He appeared malnourished. He was 180 cm (6 feet tall) and weighed

37

66 kg (146 lb). His skin was cool and clammy. The patient said, "I'm so short of breath!"

His vital signs were as follows: blood pressure 155/110, heart rate 95 bpm, respiratory rate 25/min, and oral temperature 38.3° C (101° F). He was using his accessory muscles of inspiration and pursed-lip breathing. An enlarged anteroposterior diameter of the chest was easily visible. Percussion revealed that he had low-lying hemidiaphragms. Expiration was prolonged, and his breath sounds were diminished. No wheezes were noted, but crackles could be heard over the right lower lobe.

A chest x-ray showed pulmonary hyperexpansion, severe apical pleural scarring, a large bulla in the right middle lobe, and a right lower lobe infiltrate consistent with pneumonia (Fig. 3-1). On instruction the patient's forced cough was weak and productive of a small amount of yellow sputum. On 1.5 L/min oxygen by nasal cannula, his ABGs were as follows: pH 7.59, $PaCO_2$ 40 mm Hg, HCO_3^- 37 mmol/L, and PaO_2 38 mm Hg. The physician ordered a pulmonary consult and stated that she did not want to commit the patient to a ventilator if possible. The patient also was started on intravenous doses of aminophylline and methylprednisolone.

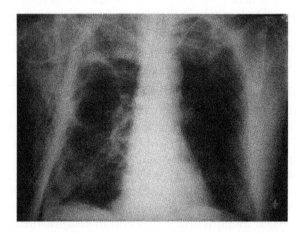

Fig. 3-1 Chest x-ray of a 62-year-old man with emphysema.

Response 1

Based on the previous information, write your SOAP in the following space.

S _____

_____

O _____

_____

_____

Response 1—cont'd

_____

_____

_____

_____

_____

A _____

_____

_____

_____

_____

_____

_____

P _____

_____

_____

_____

_____

_____

2 DAYS LATER

At this time the patient stated that his chest was feeling tighter and that he was even more short of breath. His vital signs were as follows: blood pressure 160/115, heart rate 97 bpm, respiratory rate 15/min and shallow, and oral temperature 37.8° C (100° F). Expectorated sputum was thick, yellow, and tenacious. He no longer was using his accessory muscles of inspiration or pursed-lip breathing. His breath sounds were diminished bilaterally, and crackles no longer could be heard over the right lower lobe. Dull percussion notes were elicited over the right lower lobe. His ABGs were as follows: pH 7.28, $Paco_2$ 82 mm Hg, HCO_3^- 36 mmol/L, and Pao_2 41 mm Hg. His hemoglobin oxygen saturation measured by pulse oximetry (Spo_2) was 68%. A repeat chest x-ray showed more extensive pulmonary infiltrates, particularly in the right lower chest. The physician ordered subcutaneous terbutaline every 8 hours.

Response 2

Based on the previous information, write your SOAP in the following space.

S _____

_____

O _____

_____

_____

_____

_____

_____

_____

_____

A _____

_____

_____

_____

_____

_____

_____

_____

Response 2—cont'd

P

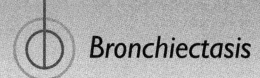

Bronchiectasis

4

ADMITTING HISTORY

A 56-year-old black woman is acquainted with the medical staff because of frequent episodes of upper respiratory infections. The woman works 40 or more hours per week as a file clerk at a local health department and is known as a hard worker. Despite what she describes as her "chronic cold," she rarely misses a day of work, although she frequently needs to request permission to leave work early because of doctor appointments. Fortunately, her immediate supervisor is a compassionate person and understands the woman's health problem and frequent requests to leave early.

The woman's hospital chart shows that her respiratory problems began when she was in her early teens. During that period, frequent upper respiratory tract infections and an annoying cough were her only symptoms. The chart also states that she was a smoker of about one pack of cigarettes per day during her teen years. Over the years she has quit and restarted smoking many times. For the past several years she has treated herself with aerosolized bronchodilators and kept a humidifier running in her room most of the time. She frequently has been given antibiotics in alternating cycles. Her husband often administers chest percussion and postural drainage at home, and she finds this treatment helpful for acute flare-ups (cough and increased sputum production).

The woman stated that she had not smoked for 3 months. Over the last 6 months, however, she stated that she had lost both weight and her generally "good spirits." She further stated that her cough was almost continuous, with production of copious amounts of foul-smelling, purulent sputum. She denied hemoptysis. She also indicated that her co-workers had become concerned about her condition and recommended that she seek immediate medical attention.

PHYSICAL EXAMINATION (TIME: 0930)

The patient appeared well-nourished and complained of severe, nearly constant shortness of breath; a frequent, strong cough; and purulent sputum production. She appeared cyanotic, and her fingers and toes showed mild clubbing. She was pursed-lip breathing and using her accessory muscles of inspiration. Coughing episodes produced large amounts of foul-smelling, yellow-green sputum.

Her vital signs were as follows: blood pressure 185/90, heart rate 110 bpm, respiratory rate 30/min, and oral temperature 37.9° C (100.2° F). Palpation of the chest and percussion of the lungs revealed no remarkable abnormalities. On auscultation, bilateral rhonchi and persistent crackles over the lung bases were heard.

Examination of her chart revealed mild-to-moderate airway obstruction on pulmonary function tests (PFTs) performed 2 years ago. Her history also showed the following baseline arterial blood gas values (ABGs) on 2 L/min oxygen: pH 7.38, $Paco_2$ 55 mm Hg, HCO_3^- 33 mmol/L, and Pao_2 68 mm Hg. On this day her bedside peak expiratory flow rate (PEFR) was 325 L/min, and her ABGs on 3 L/min O_2 by nasal cannula were as follows: pH 7.52, $Paco_2$ 35 mm Hg, HCO_3^- 27 mmol/L, and Pao_2 53 mm Hg. Her chest x-ray revealed changes suggesting cystic bronchiectasis, alveolar hyperinflation, and generalized increased bronchovascular markings (Fig. 4-1). The physician called for a respiratory care consult.

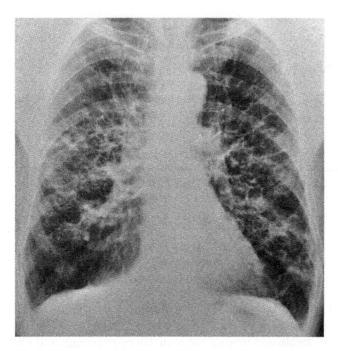

Fig. 4-1 Chest x-ray of a 56-year-old woman with bronchiectasis.

Response 1

Based on the previous information, write your SOAP in the following space.

S _____

_____

O _____

_____

Response 1—cont'd

A

P

2 DAYS AFTER ADMISSION

The woman continued to experience respiratory distress. When questioned, the patient indicated that she had felt short of breath for several hours. She appeared cyanotic, was pursed-lip breathing, and was using her accessory muscles of respiration. She continued to cough frequently and produced large amounts of foul-smelling, blood-streaked, yellow-green sputum. The sputum culture revealed *Streptococcus pneumoniae* and *Pseudomonas aeruginosa*.

Her vital signs were as follows: blood pressure 188/95, heart rate 118 bpm, respiratory rate 34/min, and oral temperature 37° C (98.6° F). Palpation of the chest was not remarkable. Percussion revealed flatness over the right lower lobe. On auscultation, bilateral rhonchi and crackles could be heard over the lung bases. Bronchial breath sounds were audible over the right lower lung base. Her oxygen saturation measured by pulse oximetry (SpO_2) was 93%. Her ABGs were as follows: pH 7.54, $PaCO_2$ 30 mm Hg, HCO_3^- 28 mmol/L, and PaO_2 57 mm Hg. A current chest x-ray revealed density in the right lower lobe that was consistent with atelectasis or acute pneumonia.

Response 2

Based on the previous information, write your SOAP in the following space.

S _____

_____

O _____

_____

_____

_____

_____

_____

_____

A _____

_____

_____

_____

_____

_____

Response 2–cont'd

P _____

4 DAYS AFTER ADMISSION

During an assessment and treatment session the patient stated that she was breathing much better. Although she was still pale, she demonstrated no remarkable cyanosis, pursed-lip breathing, or use of accessory muscles of respiration. When asked to give a strong cough, she did so and produced a moderate amount of thin, clear secretions. Her vital signs were as follows: blood pressure 135/85, heart rate 80 bpm, respiratory rate 14/min, and temperature normal. Mild rhonchi and crackles still were auscultated over the bases of both lung fields. Her SpO_2 was 94%, and her ABGs were as follows: pH 7.48, $PaCO_2$ 49 mm Hg, HCO_3^- 38 mmol/L, and PaO_2 66 mm Hg. A current chest x-ray no longer showed an opacity in the right lower lobe.

Response 3

Based on the previous information, write your SOAP in the following space.

S _____

O _____

Continued

Response 3–cont'd

A

P

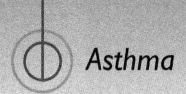

Asthma

ADMITTING HISTORY

A 10-year-old girl is well known to the respiratory care protocol team. Over the past 8 years she was hospitalized for severe asthma three or four times per year. She averaged 2- to 3-day hospital stays per admission. Over the past 4 years she required mechanical ventilation three separate times. Because of her excessive absenteeism from school, the girl was held back in the second grade. At the time of this admission the patient was in the fourth grade.

About 2 years ago the girl's mother lost her job as a teller at a local bank because of the many days she needed to take off from work to take her daughter to the doctor. For the past 15 months the mother has been able to work only part time as a checkout clerk at a local grocery store. This turn of events further compromised an already extensive and growing medical bill.

The last time the patient was on a ventilator was about 2 years ago. After that hospitalization, her mother–a single parent–quit smoking, a habit she practiced for about 20 years, and gave away the family cat. In addition, the family's mobile home and its heating system were cleaned thoroughly, and several portable air-conditioning units were installed. For the past 6 months the girl has been on an albuterol inhaler four times a day and as needed; a beclomethasone inhaler four times a day; and oral theophylline twice daily. Her mother was instructed in the proper way to monitor her daughter's peak expiratory flow rate (PEFR) regularly. The patient's personal best PEFR was about 290 L/min.

During a recent doctor's appointment, allergy skin tests turned up positive for ragweed and grasses. She was begun on a program of hyposensitization. Despite these efforts the girl still had a number of bad asthmatic episodes. Two episodes required hospitalization. Mechanical ventilation was not required in either case.

The patient was last hospitalized 6 weeks earlier. Her PEFR on admission was 175 L/min, and she had severe hypoxemia. At that time she received aerosolized albuterol almost continuously for 3 hours and oxygen therapy per protocol. The physician on duty treated her aggressively with intravenous aminophylline and steroids. The patient progressively improved. Her arterial blood gas values (ABGs) returned to normal within 6 hours of her admission. She was discharged the next afternoon. Fortunately, because the asthma episode occurred over a weekend, she did not miss any school days.

About 6 hours before the current admission the patient had gone to bed (at 9 PM) with no respiratory complaints, although she had been achy and tired for about

1 week. At approximately 1:30 AM she awoke short of breath. After alerting her mother, she took two puffs of her albuterol inhaler. The mother then measured her daughter's PEFR and noted that it was 235 L/min. Hoping that this asthma episode would subside soon, she instructed her daughter to take another puff of her inhaler. She then encouraged her daughter to try and go back to sleep.

Within 45 minutes, however, the girl's condition had not improved and in fact was becoming progressively worse. Her PEFR at this time was 210 L/min. Again the mother had her daughter take two puffs of her albuterol inhaler. Then, minutes later the mother again asked her daughter to exhale forcefully into her peak flow meter. Her PEFR was 170 L/min. At this point she put her daughter, still in her pajamas, into the car and drove to the hospital emergency room.

PHYSICAL EXAMINATION (TIME: 0315)

On admission to the emergency department the patient demonstrated extreme shortness of breath. She was sitting up with her legs crossed on the hospital gurney, her hands and arms in front of her and anchored to her knees in a tripod position. She was using her accessory muscles of inspiration and pursed-lip breathing and was crying, anxious in appearance, and cyanotic. She stated, "I feel horrible, and my chest is tight." She frequently demonstrated a strong, productive cough. Her sputum was moderate in quantity and thick and white.

Her PEFR was 150 L/min. Her heart rate was 190 bpm; her blood pressure was 110/85, and she had a respiratory rate of 28/min. Her temperature was normal. Auscultation revealed diminished breath sounds, wheezing, and rhonchi bilaterally. Her chest x-ray showed severe air trapping, with depressed hemidiaphragms and hyperlucency of the lungs (Fig. 5-1). Her hemoglobin oxygen saturation measured by pulse oximetry (SpO_2) on 2 L/min oxygen by nasal cannula was 77%, and her ABGs were as follows: pH 7.45, $PaCO_2$ 28 mm Hg, HCO_3^- 19 mmol/L, and PaO_2 40 mm Hg. The physician had the patient transferred to the pediatric intensive care unit. A respiratory care consult was requested. On the patient's chart the physician had written, "Respiratory care—please assess and treat as aggressively as our protocol boundaries permit. I want to keep this patient off the ventilator if possible."

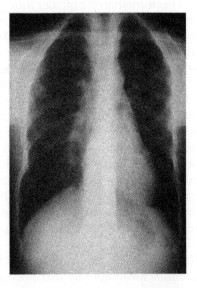

Fig. 5-1 Chest x-ray of a 10-year-old girl with asthma.

Response 1

Based on the previous information, write your SOAP in the following space.

S _____

_____

O _____

_____

_____

_____

_____

_____

_____

_____

A _____

_____

_____

_____

_____

_____

_____

_____

P _____

_____

_____

_____

_____

_____

TIME: 0530 (SAME DAY)

Since her admission, neither the patient nor her mother had been able to sleep. The patient was in a high Fowler's position, with her arms fixed to the side bedrails. She was using her accessory muscles of inspiration and pursed-lip breathing and was cyanotic. She had a frequent, strong cough that produced a moderate amount of thick, white secretions during each coughing episode. Her chest still appeared hyperinflated. She stated, "I'm sorry. I'm wheezing too much, and I can't go to sleep."

Her PEFR at this time was 175 L/min. Her heart rate was 180 bpm, blood pressure 105/82, and respiratory rate 24/min. Hyperresonant percussion notes were produced bilaterally. On auscultation, she demonstrated prolonged expiration, diminished breath sounds, rhonchi, and wheezing bilaterally. No follow-up chest x-ray had been taken. Her SpO_2 was 95%, and her ABGs were as follows: pH 7.48, $PaCO_2$ 34 mm Hg, HCO_3^- 24 mmol/L, and PaO_2 73 mm Hg.

Response 2

Based on the previous information, write your SOAP in the following space.

S _____

_____

O _____

_____

_____

_____

_____

_____

_____

_____

A _____

_____

_____

_____

Response 2–cont'd

_____

_____

_____

_____

_____

P _____

_____

_____

_____

_____

_____

TIME: 0745 (SAME DAY)

The day-shift therapist assigned to the patient gathered clinical data during her morning rounds. The patient stated that she felt as though a weight were on her chest. She was using her accessory muscles of inspiration and pursed-lip breathing. Her skin was damp and cool, and she was cyanotic. No cough or sputum production was noted. Her PEFR was 145 L/min. Her vital signs were as follows: blood pressure 160/100, heart rate 185 bpm, and respiratory rate 13/min. Her breath sounds were diminished bilaterally, and no wheezes or rhonchi were audible during auscultation. Hyperresonant percussion notes were elicited bilaterally. Her SpO_2 was 79% and her ABGs were as follows: pH 7.27, $PaCO_2$ 57 mm Hg, HCO_3^- 24 mmol/L, and PaO_2 51 mm Hg.

Response 3

Based on the previous information, write your SOAP in the following space.

S _____

_____

_____

Continued

Response 3–cont'd

O _____

_____

_____

_____

_____

_____

_____

_____

_____

A _____

_____

_____

_____

_____

_____

_____

_____

_____

_____

P _____

_____

_____

_____

_____

_____

_____

_____

KEY POINT QUESTIONS

For Asthma (DRG* 98)

1. Basic Concept Formation
   a. Are *children* affected with asthma?
   b. Are *adults* affected with asthma?
   c. Is the *cause* of asthma hyperreactivity of the airway to allergic substances?
   d. Is the *treatment* of asthma *simple?* Is it always *successful?*
   e. Are the main *clinical manifestations* of asthma cough and sputum production? If not, what are the common *clinical manifestations* of asthma?
   f. Are patients or caregivers of patients with asthma allowed to *increase or decrease their treatment* on the basis of the clinical manifestations?
   g. Which class(es) of inhaled agents do symptomatic asthmatics commonly use to treat their condition?
   h. What is the *time course* of asthma? Over hours? Over days? Over the life of the patient?
2. Database Formation
   a. What is the underlying pathophysiologic abnormality in cases of bronchial asthma?
   b. What is your *vision* of the pathologic process of bronchial asthma?
   c. What are the *various types* of asthma?
   d. Which *pathophysiologic mechanisms* are activated as a result of the typical anatomic alterations?
   e. Which portion(s) of the *airway model* (see Fig. 1-3) is/are abnormal in individuals with asthma?
   f. What are the *goals of therapy* for asthmatic patients? What constitutes *"good control"* of asthma?
   g. Which *standard modalities* should help achieve these goals?
   h. List the typical therapies ordered, expected outcomes, and monitors of each modality.
3. Assessment
   a. Did this patient initially or subsequently demonstrate any evidence of the *clinical manifestations* of bronchial asthma? If so, what were they?
   b. Did this patient initially demonstrate any evidence of the *pathophysiologic alterations* associated with bronchial asthma?
   c. Which *specific clinical manifestations* of asthma did this patient initially demonstrate that helped you determine the *severity* of her condition?
4. Application
   a. Oxygen therapy (was/was not) indicated in this patient because _____ _____ .
   b. Monitoring (was/was not) indicated because _____ .
   c. Bronchial hygiene therapy (was/was not) indicated because _____ _____ .
   d. Aerosolized medication therapy (was/was not) indicated because _____ _____ .
   e. Hyperinflation therapy (was/was not) indicated because _____ _____ .
   f. Intubation *or* mechanical ventilation (was/was not) *initially* indicated because _____ .

DRG, Diagnosis-related group.   *Continued*

KEY POINT QUESTIONS—cont'd

5. Evaluation
   a. What are the expected outcomes of each aspect of therapy you have selected?
   b. How can you *monitor* the patient's response?
   c. What are the upper limits of the *intensity or frequency* of administration of each modality?
   d. What are the *advantages* of each treatment modality?
   e. What do you do if the patient improves?
   f. What do you do if she does not?
6. Boundary Awareness
   a. How can you tell if *this* patient's condition does not improve or worsens?
   b. Can the patient or her parent or caregiver be of any help if the condition worsens?
   c. When should you ask a supervisor for help?
   d. When should you contact the patient's physician?
   e. How would you recognize actual or impending ventilatory failure in this patient?
   f. What *dangers* are present in the treatment(s) you have selected in her case?

PART III

Infectious Pulmonary Diseases

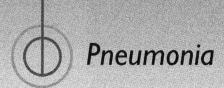

Pneumonia

ADMITTING HISTORY

A 79-year-old man was admitted to the hospital because of cough, fever, and a right lower lobe infiltrate. He was born in Detroit and worked as a truck driver for a dry-cleaning chemicals company for 51 years. He was always a hard worker and an active member of Teamsters Local 299. As a truck driver, he was often on the road 3 to 4 days at a time.

He never married, and after his sister died when he was 55 years old, he no longer had any living relatives. He started smoking at 14 years of age and averaged about two packs of cigarettes per day. When he was not working, he consumed alcohol regularly. Despite his smoking and drinking habits, he retired in good health at 65 years of age.

The patient was last admitted to the hospital 2 years ago for an acute inferior myocardial infarction. He was treated with medications and recovered quite well. He stopped smoking at that time but continued to consume alcohol regularly. He reported that he generally consumed about four to six bottles of beer each night at a local bar with some fellow retired "buddies." After his myocardial infarction he continued to manage his daily affairs without difficulty. He exercised regularly by working in his yard each day, and he power-walked every other day at the mall.

Then, 4 days before this current admission the man reported that he began experiencing "flulike" symptoms. He had chills, a mild fever, and a hacking, nonproductive cough. Although he was not feeling good, he continued to work in his yard and power-walk at the mall. He also socialized and consumed beer with his friends each night. The evening before this admission his friends noted that he was progressively getting worse and encouraged him to see a doctor. Thinking he would feel better soon, he stated that if he did not feel better in a week, he would visit his doctor. The next day, however, the patient was very short of breath, his cough was more frequent, and he had a temperature of 38.3° C (101° F). At that point he drove himself to the hospital.

PHYSICAL EXAMINATION

On inspection the patient was a well-nourished man in obvious respiratory distress on 2 L/min oxygen by nasal cannula. He was monitored by pulse oximetry. The patient stated that he was very short of breath. He had a blood pressure of 165/90, heart rate of 120 bpm, respiratory rate of 33/min, and an oral temperature of 39.5° C (103° F). He demonstrated a frequent, strong cough. His cough was "hacky" and productive of a small amount of white and yellow sputum. His skin appeared pale and damp. When the man repeated the phrase *ninety-nine,* increased tactile and vocal fremitus was noted over the right lower lung posteriorly. Dull percussion notes and bronchial breath sounds were noted over the right lower lung regions posteriorly. His oxygen saturation measured by pulse oximetry (SpO$_2$) was 87%, and his arterial blood gases (ABGs) were as follows: pH 7.56, Paco$_2$ 24 mm Hg, HCO$_3^-$ 22 mmol/L, and Pao$_2$ 56 mm Hg. His chest x-ray demonstrated a right lower lobe infiltrate consistent with pneumonia, air bronchograms, and alveolar consolidation (Fig. 6-1). His white blood cell (WBC) count was 21,000/mm^3.

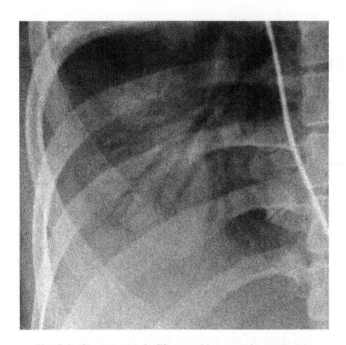

Fig. 6-1 Chest x-ray of a 79-year-old man with pneumonia.

Response 1

Based on the previous information, write your SOAP in the following space.

S _____

_____

O _____

_____

Response 1—cont'd

_____

_____

_____

_____

_____

_____

A _____

_____

_____

_____

_____

_____

P _____

_____

_____

_____

_____

_____

6 HOURS LATER

The therapist performing assessment rounds gathered the following clinical information:

The patient stated, "My doctor is too young. I feel worse than when I came in here." He had a blood pressure of 140/70, a heart rate of 125 bpm, a shallow respiratory rate of 35/min, and a temperature of 38.9° C (102° F).

He demonstrated a strong, "barking" cough, and during each major coughing episode he produced a small amount of blood-streaked sputum.

His skin appeared cyanotic. Over his right lower and middle lobes and his left lower lobe, he demonstrated increased tactile and vocal fremitus, dull percussion notes, bronchial breath sounds, and crackles. His SpO_2 was 86%. His ABGs were as follows: pH 7.55, $PaCO_2$ 26 mm Hg, HCO_3^- 24 mmol/L, and PaO_2 53 mm Hg.

Response 2

Based on the previous information, write your SOAP in the following space.

S _____

_____

O _____

_____

_____

_____

_____

_____

_____

_____

_____

A _____

_____

_____

_____

_____

_____

_____

_____

Response 2—cont'd

P _____

_____

_____

_____

_____

_____

THE NEXT DAY

The respiratory therapist assigned to evaluate the patient gathered the following clinical information:

The patient stated that he slept most of the night and was breathing easier.
The patient's blood pressure was 135/85; his heart rate was 90 bpm; his respiratory rate was 19/min; and he had an oral temperature of 37.3° C (99° F).
He had a strong, nonproductive cough.

His morning chest x-ray and report indicated partial resolution of the pneumonic process but persistent consolidation or atelectasis in the right lower and middle lobes and left lower lobe. In these lung areas the tactile and vocal fremitus had increased, and dull percussion notes and bronchial breath sounds were audible. His SpO_2 was 97%. His ABGs were as follows: pH 7.44, $PaCO_2$ 35 mm Hg, HCO_3^- 24 mmol/L, and PaO_2 163 mm Hg.

Response 3

Based on the previous information, write your SOAP in the following space.

S _____

_____

O _____

_____

Continued

Response 3−cont'd

A

P

KEY POINT QUESTIONS

For Pneumonia (DRG* 79, 89, 90)

1. Basic Concept Formation
   a. Is pneumonia an *allergic* disorder? Is it usually caused by an *infectious* agent? Is it sometimes *contagious?*
   b. Are cough and fever common *clinical manifestations* of pneumonia?
   c. Which class of drugs is almost always used in the *treatment* of pneumonia?
   d. Can pneumonia be *fatal?*
2. Database Formation
   a. What is your *vision of the pathologic process* of acute pneumonia?
   b. What are the *common causes* of pneumonia? Do they differ in different segments of the population?
   c. Which *pathophysiologic mechanisms* are activated as a result of the typical anatomic alterations?
   d. How is *severe* community-acquired pneumonia (CAP) *defined?*
   e. What are the current criteria for *hospitalization* of patients with CAP?
   f. What are the *goals of therapy* for hospitalized patients with pneumonia?
   g. Which *standard therapist-driven protocols* most likely would help achieve these goals?
   h. What are the common *complications* of pneumonia?
3. Assessment
   a. Does the patient in this case study initially or subsequently demonstrate any classic *clinical manifestations* of pneumonia? If so, what are they?
   b. Did this patient demonstrate any evidence of the *pathophysiologic abnormalities* commonly associated with acute pneumonia? If so, which ones?
   c. Which specific *clinical manifestations* of pneumonia helped you decide on the severity of his condition?
4. Application
   a. Sputum sample/induction (was/was not) indicated in this patient because _____ .
   b. Oxygen therapy (was/was not) indicated because _____ .
   c. Bronchial hygiene therapy (was/was not) indicated because _____ _____ .
   d. Aerosolized medication therapy (was/was not) indicated because _____ _____ .
   e. Hyperinflation therapy (was/was not) indicated because _____ .
5. Evaluation
   a. What are the expected outcomes of each therapeutic modality you have selected?
   b. How can you *monitor* the patient's response to therapy?
   c. What are the upper limits of the intensity of the therapy you have started on this patient?
   d. What would you do if the patient's *oxygenation worsened* or if CO_2 *retention and respiratory acidemia* occurred?
6. Boundary Awareness
   a. How can you tell if *this* patient's condition does not improve or worsens?
   b. In this case, should you have called for the supervisor after the first assessment?
   c. When should you call the physician in this case?
   d. How (did/would) you recognize impending ventilatory failure in this patient?

---

*DRG, *Diagnosis-related group.*

Human Immunodeficiency Virus (HIV)

ADMITTING HISTORY

A 26-year-old white man entered the emergency room complaining of a sore throat and persistent cough. He stated that his ability to swallow had worsened progressively over the last 2 weeks. He indicated that the pain was so severe that he was unable to eat solid food and had begun to find it difficult to swallow fluids.

Obtaining a history was difficult. The patient's answers were often vague, and he rarely looked the nurse in the eyes as he spoke. The man denied having any major medical problems. The nurse learned that about 8 months before this admission the patient had had the flu for about a week and received treatment for a rash on his back. Shortly after this period the patient recalled first noticing the irritating cough, which persisted.

The patient also has a history of a low hemoglobin level, for which he takes iron tablets. He admitted to previous intravenous drug use but stated that he has been drug free for the past 2 months. He confirmed that he has no family physician and stated that when he did become ill, he would go to various emergency rooms and clinics in the area.

The patient said that he occasionally experiences symptoms of upper respiratory tract infection, with nasal congestion and a loose cough productive of clear, white sputum. He also said that he has chills and night sweats, sometimes so severe that he has to change his clothes and bed linens. Finally, he noted that he has become increasingly tired over the past several weeks.

PHYSICAL EXAMINATION

The patient appeared pale and malnourished, sitting upright with his legs hanging over the side of the gurney and his hands and arms to his side, bracing himself on the side of the gurney. He had mild facial acne, a slight rash on his anterior chest and neck, and two herpeslike blisters on his lower lip. He stated that his throat was "killing him" and that his cough was "driving him nuts!" During the physical examination he frequently demonstrated a strong, nonproductive cough.

His vital signs were as follows: blood pressure 137/90, heart rate 95 bpm, respiratory rate 20/min, and rectal temperature 37° C (98.6° F). Lymph nodes in his neck were noted as swollen. Dull percussion notes were produced over his lung bases, and bronchial breath sounds were auscultated over the same areas. His chest x-ray showed infiltrates in both lower lung fields consistent with pneumonia (Fig. 7-1). His arterial blood gas values (ABGs) on room air were as follows: pH 7.47, $Paco_2$ 33 mm Hg, HCO_3^- 23 mmol/L, and Pao_2 76 mm Hg. His white blood cell (WBC) count was 7500. The physician called for a respiratory consult and requested an induced sputum sample for a Gram stain and sputum culture.

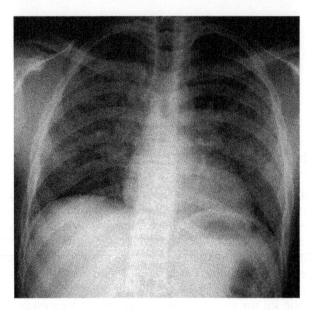

Fig. 7-1 Chest x-ray of a 26-year-old man with human immunodeficiency virus.

Response 1

Based on the previous information, write your SOAP in the following space.

S _____

_____

O _____

_____

_____

_____

_____

_____

_____

Response 1–cont'd

A _____

_____

_____

_____

_____

_____

_____

P _____

_____

_____

_____

_____

_____

3 DAYS LATER

The respiratory care practitioner found the patient lying in bed and short of breath. He stated, "I'm not breathing very well. I'm getting worse." He coughed every few minutes. The cough was strong and nonproductive. His vital signs were as follows: blood pressure 185/100, heart rate 125 bpm, respiratory rate 31/min, and rectal temperature 37° C (98.6° F). Over the right middle and lower lobes and the left lower lobe, dull percussion notes and bronchial breath sounds were noted. No recent chest x-ray was available. His oxygen saturation measured by pulse oximetry (SpO_2) was 92%, and his ABGs were as follows: pH 7.54, $PaCO_2$ 27 mm Hg, HCO_3^- 22 mmol/L, and PaO_2 54 mm Hg. A sputum culture revealed normal respiratory flora.

Response 2

Based on the previous information, write your SOAP in the following space.

S _____

_____

O _____

_____

_____

_____

_____

_____

_____

A _____

_____

_____

_____

_____

_____

_____

P _____

_____

_____

_____

_____

THE NEXT DAY

Concerned with the patient's deteriorating respiratory status, the nurse called the respiratory care consult service and requested an update. On entering the room, the respiratory therapist observed the patient to be dyspneic and in obvious respiratory distress. Although the patient was awake, he generally kept his eyes closed and merely turned his head from side to side when the therapist asked how he was feeling. No cough was noted at this time. His vital signs were as follows: blood pressure 170/85, heart rate 145 mm Hg, respiratory rate 30/min and shallow, and rectal temperature 40° C (104° F).

His morning chest x-ray showed greater infiltration and air bronchograms throughout the right middle and lower lung lobes and the left lower lung lobe. A second laboratory screening test showed that the patient's blood was positive for anti-HIV antibodies. A Western blot assay was ordered. SpO_2 was 77%, and his ABGs were as follows: pH 7.28, $PaCO_2$ 61 mm Hg, HCO_3^- 27 mmol/L, and PaO_2 47 mm Hg. The WBC count was 15,200/mm^3.

Response 3

Based on the previous information, write your SOAP in the following space.

S _____

_____

O _____

_____

_____

_____

_____

_____

_____

A _____

_____

_____

_____

Continued

Response 3—cont'd

_____

_____

_____

_____

P _____

_____

_____

_____

_____

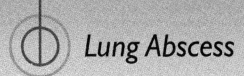

Lung Abscess

8

ADMITTING HISTORY

A 36-year-old Spanish-American woman has been homeless for the past 15 years and has lived on the streets most of that time. When the weather is very cold, she generally enters a downtown shelter. She has a history of alcohol abuse, although she did not consume alcohol during the preceding year. She is a heavy smoker and has been known to smoke up to three or four packs of cigarettes a day. Despite her rough living conditions, her personal hygiene in general appears good.

Over the past 3 years the woman has visited a physician who volunteers at the downtown clinic weekly. The entire medical staff is familiar with her condition because in the past they have treated her for her alcohol-related problems, hypothermia during one especially cold winter, numerous bouts of pneumonia, and various scrapes, cuts, and broken bones caused by frequent falls. Before visiting the health clinic this time, however, the woman had seemed better and even indicated that she had assumed a better outlook on life. On this day, though, the physician was concerned to see the patient back at the clinic and looking poorly.

PHYSICAL EXAMINATION

On physical examination the patient appeared thin and undernourished, with a disheveled appearance. She was sitting in the upright position and leaning forward on the bedside table. The patient said, "I spit all the time." She was cyanotic, and her teeth and mouth were in especially poor condition. She had a weak-to-moderate, frequent cough productive of foul-smelling, purulent sputum. After each coughing episode she wiped her mouth and nose with her sleeve.

Even though she did not appear intoxicated, her speech was nearly unintelligible, and she was confused. Her skin was dirty, and several bruises could be seen on her arms and legs. The patient's friend gave a history that the patient had been losing weight, appeared tired all the time, and had felt excessively warm to the touch for the preceding week.

Her vital signs were as follows: blood pressure 145/75, heart rate 110 bpm, respiratory rate 33/min, and oral temperature 39.3° C (102.8° F). Mild digital cyanosis was noted. Auscultation revealed crackles and rhonchi over the right middle and lower lung lobes. Normal vesicular breath sounds were heard over the left lung.

Tactile and vocal fremitus were noted over the right lung. Her arterial blood gas values (ABGs) on 2 L/min oxygen by nasal cannula were as follows: pH 7.49, $PaCO_2$ 30 mm Hg, HCO_3^- 22 mmol/L, and PaO_2 63 mm Hg. Her chest x-ray revealed a partially fluid-filled, 10-cm cavity in the right upper lobe and increased opacity in both the middle and right upper lobes (Fig. 8-1).

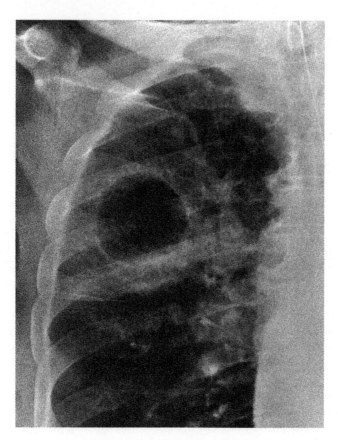

Fig. 8-1 Chest x-ray of a 36-year-old woman with a lung abscess.

Response 1

Based on the previous information, write your SOAP in the following space.

S _____

_____

O _____

_____

_____

Response 1–cont'd

A _____

P _____

24 HOURS LATER

During morning rounds the respiratory care practitioner working on the consult team noted that the patient still had a frequent, weak cough and continued to expectorate thick, purulent sputum. The patient stated, however, that she did not feel as short of breath as she had the day before. Overall, she appeared better and more alert and she was not cyanotic. Compared with the day before, her speech was more intelligible.

Her vital signs were as follows: blood pressure 135/80, heart rate 98 bpm, respiratory rate 20/min, and oral temperature 37.9° C (100.2° F). (She was currently on aspirin.) Over the right middle and lower lobes, tactile and vocal fremitus were documented, and crackles and rhonchi were heard on auscultation. Her ABGs were as follows: pH 7.48, $Paco_2$ 34 mm Hg, HCO_3^- 23 mmol/L, and Pao_2 81 mm Hg. Her hemoglobin oxygen saturation measured by pulse oximetry (Spo_2) was 96%. No chest x-ray had been ordered for the day.

Response 2

Based on the previous information, write your SOAP in the following space.

S _____

_____

O _____

_____

_____

_____

_____

_____

_____

A _____

_____

_____

_____

_____

_____

_____

Response 2–cont'd

P _____

_____

_____

_____

_____

_____

3 DAYS LATER

At this time the patient stated, "You doctors cured my damn cough!" The patient's skin no longer appeared cyanotic, and no spontaneous cough was noted. When asked to force a cough, the patient produced a strong cough, but no sputum production was noted. Her vital signs were as follows: blood pressure 127/82, heart rate 86 bpm, respiratory rate 16/min, and oral temperature 36.8° C (98.2° F).

No tactile or vocal fremitus was detected over the right middle and upper lobes. Crackles, however, still could be auscultated over the right lower lobe. Her ABGs were as follows: pH 7.43, $PaCO_2$ 36 mm Hg, HCO_3^- 24 mmol/L, and PaO_2 163 mm Hg. Her SpO_2 was 97%. Although the morning chest x-ray still revealed the partially fluid-filled abscess, the infiltrate in the right middle lung lobe was improved. Some infiltrate still was seen around the abscess in the right upper lobe.

Response 3

Based on the previous information, write your SOAP in the following space.

S _____

_____

O _____

_____

_____

Continued

Response 3—cont'd

_____
_____
_____
_____
_____
_____

A _____
_____
_____
_____
_____
_____
_____
_____

P _____
_____
_____
_____
_____
_____

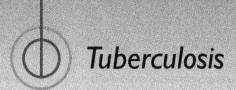

Tuberculosis

ADMITTING HISTORY

A 58-year-old white man is well known and liked by the staff at the Samaritan Shelter for the Homeless. The social workers at the shelter have spent a great deal of time and resources working with the man on a number of areas, including his alcohol addiction. Their records show that they have not seen him for about 6 months. When they last saw him, he was not drinking, had just secured a job as a janitor at a large department store, and was making enough money to eat and pay the rent on a small apartment.

The staff members were saddened when he came to the shelter in search of some food and a bed. The man appeared tired, dirty, and depressed. He smelled of alcohol. He stated that he had quit his job about 3 months previously because his boss was "a jerk." He also confirmed that he had been living on the streets again because of his inability to pay the rent. Although he chain-smoked as he talked to the staff members, he frequently complained about his "smoker's cough."

Two days after he arrived at the shelter the man began having episodes of coughing that were more severe than usual. On several occasions the coughing spells lasted more than 2 hours. Hemoptysis often occurred during these periods. When the staff members at the shelter noted that the man had expectorated about a pint of fresh blood, they decided to transfer him to the local charity hospital. Although the man initially resisted, he finally agreed to go to the hospital.

PHYSICAL EXAMINATION

In the emergency room the man appeared anxious, chronically and acutely malnourished, weak, and in obvious respiratory distress. His nail beds were cyanotic, and his fingers were yellow from nicotine stains. The patient stated that he had smoked approximately 30 cigarettes a day for 35 years. He had a frequent, strong cough, producing moderate amounts of yellow sputum mixed with small amounts of fresh blood. He stated that his cough has been getting worse, and he thought that he probably had a "cold." He also indicated that he could not seem to get his breath.

The patient denied having any respiratory problems before this admission. However, he also stated that coughing up blood was "no big deal" because he had done it a couple of times before. Although the patient denied having used alcohol for months, the staff members from the shelter documented the smell of alcohol at the time of his admission at the shelter. The patient obviously had fallen in the recent past. He had several large bruises on his forehead, on his right shoulder and arm, and over his right anterior axillary chest region, between the sixth and ninth ribs.

The patient's vital signs were as follows: blood pressure 170/95, heart rate 110 bpm, respiratory rate 26/min, and oral temperature 38.3° C (101° F). Although palpation of the chest was negative, dull percussion notes and increased tactile and vocal fremitus were noted over the lung bases. Bronchial breath sounds were heard over the right and left lung bases. Crackles and rhonchi were noted over the right upper lobe. A pleural friction rub also was auscultated over the right lower lobe, between the fifth and sixth ribs in the anterior axillary line.

A chest x-ray revealed an increased opacity consistent with pneumonia and atelectasis in the left lower lobe and right middle and upper lobes. A 5-cm cavity was easily visible in the left upper lobe (Fig. 9-1). The patient had a hemoglobin level of 17 g/dl and a white blood cell (WBC) count of 14,000/mm³. While the patient was in the emergency room, the nurse administered a Mantoux tuberculin skin test. The patient's arterial blood gas values (ABGs) on room air were as follows: pH 7.53, $PaCO_2$ 51 mm Hg, HCO_3^- 41 mmol/L, and PaO_2 50 mm Hg. His carboxyhemoglobin level was 8.5%, and his hemoglobin oxygen saturation measured by pulse oximetry (SpO_2) was 88%.

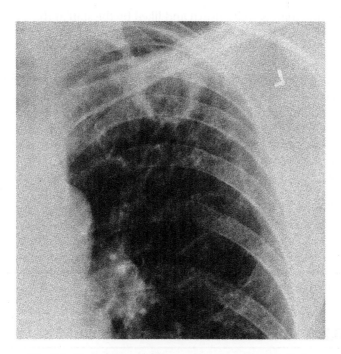

Fig. 9-1 Chest x-ray of a 58-year-old man with tuberculosis.

Response 1

Based on the previous information, write your SOAP in the following space.

S _____

_____

Response 1—cont'd

O

A

P

4 DAYS AFTER ADMISSION

In reviewing the patient's chart the respiratory care practitioner noted that the patient had a positive tuberculin reaction. An acid-fast stain and sputum culture had been obtained. Also noted was that the patient had undergone fiberoptic bronchoscopy. During this procedure, both old blood and fresh blood were found throughout the tracheobronchial tree. Secretions obtained from the large airways were negative for malignant cells.

A complete pulmonary function test (PFT) indicated a moderate-to-severe restrictive disorder. The morning chest x-ray showed an improvement in the aeration of the lung bases, as compared with the admission radiograph. The patient's cyanosis and respiratory distress appeared better. His cough was still frequent and productive. The amount of sputum, however, was not as great as that on admission. Although the sputum was opaque, it was no longer yellow, and no blood could be seen. The patient stated that his cough was a lot better.

His vital signs were as follows: blood pressure 143/90, heart rate 92 bpm, respiratory rate 18/min, and oral temperature 37.4° C (99.3° F). Dull percussion notes and bronchial breath sounds were noted over the lung bases. Rhonchi still could be heard over the right middle lobe, although they were not so pronounced as on admission. The pleural friction rub no longer was present. The patient's ABGs were as follows: pH 7.48, $Paco_2$ 60 mm Hg, HCO_3^- 42 mmol/L, and Pao_2 61 mm Hg. His Spo_2 was 91%. Acid-fast organisms were seen on direct smear of the bronchoscopically obtained secretions.

Response 2

Based on the previous information, write your SOAP in the following space.

S _____

_____

O _____

_____

_____

_____

_____

_____

_____

_____

Response 2–cont'd

A _____

_____

_____

_____

_____

_____

_____

_____

_____

P _____

_____

_____

_____

_____

_____

_____

7 DAYS AFTER ADMISSION

As part of the discharge team on this day, the respiratory care practitioner reviewed the patient's chart and noted that his morning chest x-ray had improved significantly. The parenchymal densities present in the lung bases on admission were much improved. The large cavity in the upper left lung lobe, however, was still clearly visible. While in the hospital, the patient had been started on daily doses of isoniazid and rifampin (Rifadin). Arrangements had been made with the staff at the Samaritan Shelter to dispense the prescribed drugs and monitor the patient's compliance in taking them.

On observation, the patient still appeared moderately pale and cyanotic, but he no longer appeared to be in respiratory distress. In addition, he no longer demonstrated a spontaneous, uncontrolled cough. The patient stated that he was ready to run a marathon. When asked to cough, the patient generated a strong, nonproductive cough. His vital signs were as follows: blood pressure 135/85, heart rate 80 bpm, respiratory rate 10/min, and oral temperature 37° C (98.6° F). Palpation and percussion were essentially negative. Normal vesicular breath sounds were audible over the lower lung fields. On a 1 L/min oxygen nasal cannula the patient's ABGs were as follows: pH 7.42, $Paco_2$ 72 mm Hg, HCO_3^- 45 mmol/L, and Pao_2 78 mm Hg. His Spo_2 was 94%. Three successive sputum smears over the last 4 days were acid-fast bacilli (AFB) negative.

Response 3

Based on the previous information, write your SOAP in the following space.

S _____

_____

O _____

_____

_____

_____

_____

_____

_____

_____

_____

A _____

_____

_____

_____

_____

_____

_____

_____

Response 3–cont'd

P

Fungal Diseases of the Lungs

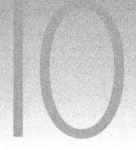

ADMITTING HISTORY

A 56-year-old cattle driver was admitted to the arthritis clinic of a small hospital just outside Phoenix because of joint pain. The man stated that the tenderness in his joints prevented him from riding his horse for any extended period. He was born on a cattle ranch in New Mexico and spent most of his adult life working as a cattle driver in Arizona, New Mexico, and Colorado. He had always considered himself an "outdoors" kind of man. He loved the range, wide open spaces, clear air, and beauty of the desert.

In his early 20s he traveled to the East Coast to attend college. While there, he became withdrawn and depressed and felt confined. After 1 year he dropped out of college and returned to New Mexico. Shortly after returning home, his symptoms of depression disappeared. He worked on a large cattle ranch, made several new friends, and was content with the fact that he "belonged on the open range." He never married or settled down in one place he could call home. He often said that the great outdoors was his home. He never owned an automobile. In fact, he often said that the only things of real value he owned were a roan quarter horse and a saddle.

The hospital had no past medical record on the patient. The man reported, however, that although he was rarely ill, he had gone to see a doctor while in Colorado about a year ago for severe "cold" symptoms, which included fever, cough, chest pain, headaches, and a general feeling of fatigue. He was a nonsmoker, although he did chew tobacco for a short time in his teens. The patient verified that he consumed alcohol regularly on Friday and Saturday nights. On average the man estimated that he consumed between 6 and 10 beers per outing and sometimes more. Despite the patient's somewhat rugged living conditions and alcohol consumption, he was not overweight and was in reasonably good physical condition.

PHYSICAL EXAMINATION

The patient appeared to be a well-developed, well-nourished white man in moderate respiratory distress. He complained of soreness and stiffness in all his joints. He also stated that he thought he had a "bad cold" and that he was short of breath.

The patient's knees and ankle joints were warm, swollen, and tender to the touch. Although his skin appeared weathered and tan, his lips and nail beds were cyanotic.

He demonstrated a frequent cough productive of a moderate amount of thick, yellow sputum. Although the cough was strong, he experienced difficulty raising sputum during each coughing episode. His vital signs were as follows: blood pressure 160/90, heart rate 93 bpm, respiratory rate 18/min, and oral temperature 37.8° C (100° F). Palpation revealed a few erythematous lesions on his anterior chest, of which he was unaware. In addition, a walnut-size erythematous lesion was present on the patient's left cheek. Percussion of the chest was not remarkable. Auscultation revealed bilateral crackles and rhonchi in the lung apices.

The patient's chest x-ray showed scattered infiltrates consistent with fibrosis and calcification and multiple spherical nodules throughout both lungs. In the upper lobes of both lungs, two to three small, 1- to 3-cm cavities were visible (Fig. 10-1). On room air the patient's arterial blood gas values (ABGs) were as follows: pH 7.51, $Paco_2$ 29 mm Hg, HCO_3^- 22 mmol/L, and Pao_2 64 mm Hg. Concerned about the patient's respiratory status, the physician requested a respiratory care consult.

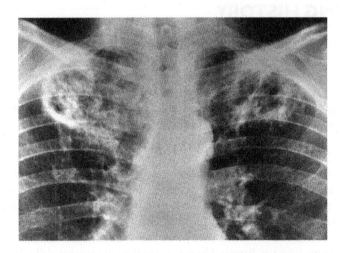

Fig. 10-1 Chest x-ray of a 56-year-old man with a fungal disease of the lungs.

Response 1

Based on the previous information, write your SOAP in the following space.

S _____

_____

O _____

_____

_____

Response 1–cont'd

A

P

5 DAYS AFTER ADMISSION

The respiratory care practitioner working with the patient at this time gathered the following clinical information from the patient's chart:

Based on microscopy of the patient's sputum and a spherulin skin test, the diagnosis of coccidioidomycosis was now written in the patient's chart.

The patient had been receiving amphotericin B intravenously for 2 days.

A complete pulmonary function study revealed a moderate-to-severe restrictive disorder, with a moderate obstructive component as well.

When the practitioner entered the patient's room, the man was sitting up in bed, appearing cyanotic, short of breath, and fatigued. He stated that he was becoming tired of people in white outfits coming in and out of his room, day and night, with needles, pills, and bills. He further stated that he still could not get a good breath of air. In fact, he said it was more difficult for him to breathe today than it had been on the day he entered the hospital.

The patient still had a frequent, strong cough productive of moderate amounts of thick, opaque sputum. His vital signs were as follows: blood pressure 165/95, heart rate 97 bpm, respiratory rate 24/min, and temperature 37° C (98.6° F). Auscultation revealed persistent bilateral tight wheezes, bilateral crackles and rhonchi in the apices of both lungs. A current chest x-ray was not available. His hemoglobin oxygen saturation measured by pulse oximetry (SpO_2) was 88%. His ABGs were as follows: pH 7.54, $PaCO_2$ 27 mm Hg, HCO_3^- 21 mmol/L, and PaO_2 55 mm Hg.

Response 2

Based on the previous information, write your SOAP in the following space.

S _____

_____

O _____

_____

_____

_____

_____

_____

_____

Response 2–cont'd

A _____

P _____

10 DAYS AFTER ADMISSION

On this day the respiratory therapist found the patient walking up and down the corridor talking to various staff members and patients. The man appeared to be in no respiratory distress. He stated that he was breathing much better and was ready to ride his horse a long distance in any direction away from the hospital.

No spontaneous cough was noted. When asked to generate a cough, the patient produced a strong, nonproductive cough. His vital signs were as follows: blood pressure 135/88, heart rate 80 bpm, respiratory rate 14/min, and normal temperature. Auscultation revealed persistent bilateral crackles in the apices of both lungs. A recent chest x-ray was not available. His pulse oximetry on room air showed an SpO_2 of 91%. His ABGs were as follows: pH 7.44, $PaCO_2$ 34 mm Hg, HCO_3^- 23 mmol/L, and PaO_2 71 mm Hg.

Response 3

Based on the previous information, write your SOAP in the following space.

S _____

_____

O _____

_____

_____

_____

_____

_____

_____

A _____

_____

_____

_____

_____

_____

_____

_____

P _____

_____

_____

_____

_____

PART IV

Pulmonary Vascular Diseases

Pulmonary Edema

ADMITTING HISTORY

A 68-year-old hypertensive man arrived in the emergency department via ambulance at 6:45 AM. The patient's wife stated that her husband had been doing well until the evening before admission, when he complained of being tired and short of breath. She also noted that he had demonstrated a sudden onset of dry, nonproductive cough. Thinking that he was getting a "touch of the flu," she gave her husband some hot soup, two aspirins, and a tablespoon of Robitussin and made him go to bed at about 8:30 PM. She stated that she had awoken about 4:30 AM to find her husband sitting up in bed, gasping for air. Alarmed, she had called 911.

The man's history shows that he had been in fairly good health since his retirement as a plumber 2 years ago. He has smoked about one pack of cigarettes a day for the past 40 years. For the past 2 years he and his wife have actively devoted most of their time to gardening and travel. They are planning a cross-country trailer trip to Alaska. About 1 year ago the man underwent a physical examination in preparation for this trip. At that time his physician placed him on digoxin and furosemide (Lasix) to treat atrial fibrillation and mild congestive heart failure, and the man quit smoking.

On the patient's arrival at the treatment room the emergency room nurse immediately placed him in a high Fowler's position. The respiratory therapist started oxygen at 2 L/min by nasal cannula. His wife appeared anxious. She was sobbing and walking back and forth, stating repeatedly, "Bill takes a heart pill and a water pill, and he follows a low-salt diet—just like the doctor told him to do."

PHYSICAL EXAMINATION (TIME: 0700)

On inspection the patient was in obvious respiratory distress. The man stated, however, "I don't think I'm having a serious problem." He further stated, "My wife and I are only 2 days away from our dream trip to Alaska. We've been planning this trip for 8 years! I can't believe this! . . . It is just 2 days before we are supposed to leave, and here I am on this emergency room gurney!"

His vital signs were as follows: blood pressure 100/50, heart rate 145 bpm and irregular, and respiratory rate 22/min. The man was afebrile. His throat was reddened. On 2 L/min oxygen, his oxygen saturation measured by pulse oximetry (SpO_2) was 70%. His lips were blue, his neck veins were distended, he appeared very anxious, and he was coughing frequently, producing small amounts of frothy, pink secretions. His abdomen was distended, and pitting edema was present to the mid-calf area. Palpation of his chest was unremarkable. Dull percussion notes were elicited over the lower lung regions bilaterally. Auscultation revealed inspiratory crackles and expiratory wheezing over the left and right lower lung regions.

His arterial blood gases (ABGs) on 2 L/min oxygen by nasal cannula were as follows: pH 7.56, $PaCO_2$ 28 mm Hg, HCO_3^- 20 mmol/L, and PaO_2 51 mm Hg. According to the radiologist's report, his chest x-ray showed faint opacities over the lower lung areas bilaterally. The x-ray report also noted that the patient's heart was moderately enlarged, suggesting left ventricular hypertrophy (Fig. 11-1).

The emergency room physician started the patient on intravenous digitalis, dobutamine, and furosemide. The physician ordered another chest x-ray film and asked the respiratory care consult service to see the patient. He specifically requested that respiratory care personnel monitor the patient closely over the next several hours.

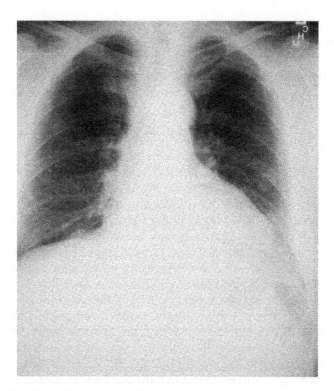

Fig. 11-1 Chest x-ray of a 68-year-old man with pulmonary edema.

Response 1

Based on the previous information, write your SOAP in the following space.

S

Response 1—cont'd

O _____

_____

_____

_____

_____

_____

_____

_____

A _____

_____

_____

_____

_____

_____

_____

_____

_____

_____

P _____

_____

_____

_____

_____

_____

_____

_____

_____

TIME: 1100

The repeat bedside chest x-ray showed no remarkable improvement. The patient stated, "I still don't feel great." His vital signs were as follows: blood pressure 160/90, heart rate 105 bpm and regular rhythm, respiratory rate 20/min, and temperature 37.1° C (98.8° F). The color of his lips had improved slightly, but no improvement was apparent in the patient's distended neck veins. The nurse noted that the man's urine output over the past 2 hours had been 650 ml. The patient still coughed frequently; however, no frothy, pink sputum was noted at this time. Auscultation continued to reveal inspiratory crackles and expiratory wheezing over the lower lung lobes bilaterally. His SpO_2 was 84%. His ABG study revealed a pH 7.54, $PaCO_2$ 25 mm Hg, HCO_3^- 18 mmol/L, and PaO_2 51 mm Hg. Neither his cardiac enzymes nor his troponin levels had risen.

Response 2

Based on the previous information, write your SOAP in the following space.

S _____

_____

O _____

_____

_____

_____

_____

_____

_____

A _____

_____

_____

_____

_____

_____

Response 2–cont'd

P

TIME: 1630

The man stated that he was breathing better. His vital signs were as follows: blood pressure 140/115, heart rate 95 bpm and regular, respiratory rate 16/min, and oral temperature 37.3° C (99.1° F). His lips and fingertips were no longer blue. The nursing chart showed that the patient's urine output over the past 2 hours had been 850 ml. The man appeared relaxed and no longer demonstrated any significant venous distension. On request the patient produced a strong, nonproductive cough. Auscultation revealed bilateral crackles over the lower lung lobes. His pulse oximetry showed an SpO_2 of 97%, and repeated ABGs were as follows: pH 7.44, $PaCO_2$ 36 mm Hg, HCO_3^- 24 mmol/L, and PaO_2 190 mm Hg.

Response 3

Based on the previous information, write your SOAP in the following space.

S

O

Continued

Response 3—cont'd

A

P

KEY POINT QUESTIONS

For Pulmonary Edema (DRG* 87)

1. Basic Concept Formation
   a. Is *heart failure* associated with dyspnea?
   b. What happens to *pulmonary venous pressure* if the *left ventricle fails?*
   c. What is the meaning of *edema?*
   d. Are the *risk factors* for heart disease and lung disease similar?
2. Database Formation
   a. What is your *vision of the pathologic process* of acute pulmonary edema?
   b. Which *pathophysiologic mechanisms* are activated as a result of these anatomic alterations?
   c. Which *clinical manifestations* might be observed if these pathophysiologic mechanisms were activated?
   d. What *other signs and symptoms* might be seen in cases of pulmonary edema?
   e. What should be the *goals of therapy* in such patients?
   f. Which *standard therapist-driven protocols* might achieve these goals?
   g. List the *outcomes* and potential *adverse effects* of each protocol you have selected and describe the way you would *monitor* their beneficial and adverse effects.
3. Assessment
   a. Did the patient in this case study demonstrate any *risk factors* for cardiac disease and congestive heart failure?
   b. Did this patient initially or subsequently demonstrate any *clinical manifestations* of acute pulmonary edema? What were they?
   c. Did the patient in this case study initially demonstrate any evidence of the *pathophysiologic alterations* typically associated with pulmonary edema? What were they?
   d. Which *specific clinical manifestations* did this patient demonstrate that helped you decide on the *severity* of his condition?
4. Application
   a. Oxygen therapy (was/was not) indicated because _____ .
   b. Monitoring (was/was not) indicated because _____ .
   c. Bronchial hygiene therapy (was/was not) indicated because _____
   _____ .
   d. Aerosolized medication therapy (was/was not) indicated because _____
   _____ .
   e. Hyperinflation therapy (was/was not) indicated because _____
   _____ .
   f. Mechanical ventilation (was/was not) indicated because _____
   _____ .
5. Evaluation
   a. What are the expected *results* of each modality or protocol you selected?
   b. How should you *monitor* the patient's response to these therapies?
   c. How much can you increase or decrease the *intensity* or *frequency* of each modality as needed?
   d. What are the *advantages and disadvantages* of each treatment modality?
   e. How should you *reduce therapy* in this case *if the patient improves?*

---

*DRG, Diagnosis-related group.

Continued

KEY POINT QUESTIONS—cont'd

6. Boundary Awareness
   a. How would you know if this patient's condition does not improve or actually worsens?
   b. When should you ask a supervisor for help?
   c. When should you call the patient's physician?
   d. How would you recognize actual or impending respiratory failure in this patient?
   e. What dangers are present in the treatments you have selected?

Pulmonary Embolism

ADMITTING HISTORY

A 32-year-old motorcycle enthusiast who smokes one pack of cigarettes per day fell asleep and fell off his bike while riding with a group of Harley "hogs" to the annual Sturgis Rally in North Dakota. Although his motorcycle sustained extensive damage, the man was conscious when the ambulance arrived. Before he was transported to the local hospital, he was treated in the field; splints and an immobilizer were applied. His injuries were thought to include a fractured pelvis, left tibia, and left knee.

En route to the hospital a partial rebreathing oxygen mask was placed over the man's face. An intravenous infusion was started with 5% glucose solution. The patient was alert and able to answer questions. His vital signs were as follows: blood pressure 150/90, heart rate 105 bpm, and respiratory rate 20/min. Various small lacerations and scrapes on his face and left shoulder were treated. Each time the man was moved slightly or when the ambulance suddenly bounced or turned sharply as it moved over the highway, he complained of abdominal and bilateral chest pain. The emergency medical technician (EMT) crew all thought that his helmet and his youth had saved his life.

In the emergency room a laboratory technician drew the patient's blood; several x-rays were taken with a portable machine, and the man was given morphine for the pain. Within an hour the patient was taken to surgery to have the broken bones in his left leg repaired. He was transferred 4 hours later to the intensive care unit (ICU) with his left leg in a cast. Thrombosis and embolism prophylaxis had been started with low-dose heparin. Busy with another surgery, the physician ordered a respiratory care consult for the patient.

PHYSICAL EXAMINATION

The respiratory therapist found the patient lying in bed with his left leg suspended about 25 cm (10 inches) above the bed surface. He had a partial rebreathing oxygen mask on his face and was alert. His wife and two young boys, who were 10 years of age and wearing black motorcycle jackets, were at the man's bedside. The patient stated that he was feeling much better and that his breathing was OK.

His vital signs were as follows: blood pressure 115/75, heart rate 75 bpm, and respiratory rate 11/min. He was afebrile, and his skin color appeared good. No remarkable breathing problems were noted. Palpation revealed mild tenderness over the left shoulder and left anterior chest area. Percussion was unremarkable, and auscultation revealed normal vesicular breath sounds. The chest x-ray taken earlier that morning in the emergency room was normal. His arterial blood gas values (ABGs) on a partial rebreathing mask were as follows: pH 7.40, $PaCO_2$ 41 mm Hg, HCO_3^- 24 mmol/L, and PaO_2 504 mm Hg. His hemoglobin oxygen saturation measured by pulse oximetry (SpO_2) was 97%.

Response 1

Based on the previous information, write your SOAP in the following space.

S _____

_____

O _____

_____

_____

_____

_____

_____

_____

_____

A _____

_____

_____

_____

_____

_____

_____

_____

Response 1–cont'd

P _____

_____

_____

_____

_____

_____

_____

3 DAYS AFTER ADMISSION

The man's general course of recovery was uneventful until the third day after his admission, when the nurses noticed swelling of the left calf while giving him a bath. A Doppler venogram revealed a left tibial deep vein thrombosis. The physician was informed. Anticoagulant therapy was started. Then, 5 hours later the patient became short of breath and agitated. A spontaneous cough was noted, productive of a small amount of blood-tinged sputum. Concerned, the nurse called the physician and respiratory care.

When the respiratory care practitioner walked into the patient's room, the man appeared cyanotic, was very short of breath, and stated that he felt awful. The patient further said that he had precordial chest pain, felt lightheaded, and had a feeling of impending doom. His vital signs were as follows: blood pressure 90/45, heart rate 125 bpm, respiratory rate 30/min, and oral temperature 37.2° C (99° F). Palpation and percussion of the chest were unremarkable. Auscultation revealed faint wheezing throughout both lung fields. A pleural friction rub was audible anteriorly over the right middle lobe. A pulmonary artery catheter had been inserted.

The patient's electrocardiographic (ECG) pattern alternated among a normal sinus rhythm, sinus tachycardia, and atrial flutter. His hemodynamic indices showed an increased central venous pressure (CVP), right atrial pressure (RAP), mean pulmonary artery pressure ($\overline{PA}$), right ventricular stroke work index (RVSWI), and pulmonary vascular resistance (PVR), as well as a decreased pulmonary capillary wedge pressure (PCWP), cardiac output (CO), stroke volume (SV), stroke volume index (SVI), and cardiac index (CI). The chest x-ray showed increased density in the right middle lobe consistent with atelectasis and consolidation. The ABGs were as follows: pH 7.53, $PaCO_2$ 26 mm Hg, HCO_3^- 21 mmol/L, and PaO_2 53 mm Hg. His SpO_2 was 89%. The physician started the patient on intravenous streptokinase, ordered a ventilation-perfusion lung scan, and requested that respiratory care see the patient again.

Response 2

Based on the previous information, write your SOAP in the following space.

S _____

_____

O _____

_____

_____

_____

_____

_____

_____

A _____

_____

_____

_____

_____

_____

_____

P _____

_____

_____

_____

_____

_____

2 HOURS LATER

The ventilation-perfusion scan showed no blood flow to the right middle lobe. The patient's eyes were closed, and he no longer was responsive to questions. His skin appeared cyanotic, and his cough was productive of a small amount of blood-tinged sputum. His vital signs were as follows: blood pressure 70/35, heart rate 160 bpm, respiratory rate 25/min and shallow, and rectal temperature 37.5° C (99.2° F). Palpation of the chest was normal. Dull percussion notes were elicited over the right midlung. Wheezing was heard throughout both lung fields, and a pleural friction rub was audible over the right middle lobe.

The patient demonstrated an ECG pattern that alternated among a normal sinus rhythm, sinus tachycardia, and atrial flutter. His hemodynamic indices continued to show an increased CVP, RAP, $\overline{PA}$, RVSWI, and PVR and a decreased PCWP, CO, SV, SVI, and CI. The patient's ABGs were as follows: pH 7.25, $Paco_2$ 69 mm Hg, HCO_3^- 27 mmol/L, and Pao_2 37 mm Hg. His Spo_2 was 64%.

Response 3

Based on the previous information, write your SOAP in the following space.

S _____

_____

O _____

_____

_____

_____

_____

_____

_____

A _____

_____

_____

_____

Continued

Response 3—cont'd

P

PART V

Chest and Pleural Trauma

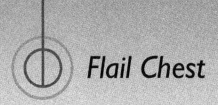

Flail Chest

ADMITTING HISTORY

A 22-year-old white man has a long history of alcohol abuse. While in middle school, he and his friends stole their parents' beer and drank regularly. By the time he was a senior in high school, he was drinking beer and Jack Daniel's whiskey almost daily. He often became mean when he was drinking and got into fights. Although he was well built and was considered nice looking, he generally could not maintain a long-term relationship with the girls he dated in high school. At graduation, however, he was dating a girl whom he married 7 months later.

The marriage was a stormy one. His wife was well known to the social workers answering the hot-line phones at the local crisis center. On several occasions his wife called the police to their mobile home with reports of spousal abuse. One time the man waved a small handgun at her and accidentally shot a hole through their kitchen wall. He always apologized extensively to his wife after a major incident and promised, to no avail, to stop drinking.

Within 1 year of their marriage he lost his job as a carpenter for missing too much work. Then, 15 months after their wedding his wife had him served with a restraining order, filed for a divorce, and moved in with her parents. He continued to drink heavily as he worked various minimum-wage jobs for the next 2 years. The local union laid him off 3 months ago for the winter season from his position as an unskilled laborer. With his unemployment checks he spent most of his days and evenings in local bars drinking, playing cards, and shooting pool. He lost his driver's license 5 weeks before this admission for a year for hitting—and totaling—a parked car while driving under the influence of alcohol.

On the day of this admission the man started drinking heavily around 4 PM. By 11:30 PM he was at a local dance club and extremely intoxicated. He was using foul language, bumping into people, yelling insults at the band, and constantly trying to start a fight with the other customers. The bouncer quickly ushered him off the premises.

The weather was bad on this night. It was cold, raining, sleeting, and dark as he walked and hitchhiked along a country road. He stumbled and staggered into the road as he walked and yelled profanities at the cars as they drove past. A witness later told the police that he appeared to dare the cars to hit him. Approximately 20 minutes after he was ejected from the dance club, he was hit by a pickup truck. The ambulance crew found him 35 yards from the road, lying in a corn field.

PHYSICAL EXAMINATION

When the man was brought into the emergency room, he was unconscious but breathing on his own through a nonrebreathing mask. He had numerous scrapes and lacerations on his face, anterior chest, and legs. Both his upper and lower front teeth were broken at the gum lines. Paradoxical movement could clearly be seen over most of his anterior chest. His skin appeared pale and cyanotic, and the smell of alcohol radiated strongly from his body. His blood alcohol level was 0.34%.

The man's vital signs were as follows: blood pressure 165/92, heart rate 120 bpm, respiratory rate 26/min and shallow, and rectal temperature 36.2° C (97.2° F). His weight was approximately 86 kg (190 lb). Breath sounds were diminished bilaterally. A chest x-ray showed extensive multiple double rib fractures of the right and left anterior and lateral ribs, between ribs 4 and 9. No pneumothorax was visible. His sternum was fractured in three separate places. Increased densities, consistent with atelectasis, were visible throughout both lung fields in the chest x-ray (Fig. 13-1). The patient's arterial blood gas values (ABGs) were as follows: pH 7.17, $Paco_2$ 82 mm Hg, HCO_3^- 27 mmol/L, and Pao_2 37 mm Hg. His oxygen saturation measured by pulse oximetry (Spo_2) was 59%.

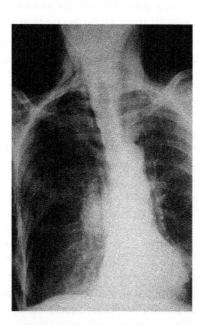

Fig. 13-1 Chest x-ray of a 22-year-old man with flail chest.

Response 1

Based on the previous information, write your SOAP in the following space.

S _____

_____

Response 1—cont'd

O

A

P

24 HOURS AFTER ADMISSION

The patient's condition was still classified as serious and unstable. He was on a mechanical ventilator in the controlled mode. A pulmonary artery catheter, a central venous pressure catheter, and an arterial line were in place. Although the patient drifted in and out of consciousness, he was on a pancuronium (Pavulon) drip and was unable to move. No paradoxical movement of the chest was detected.

His skin still appeared pale and cyanotic, and his neck veins were distended. The patient's vital signs were as follows: blood pressure 100/65, heart rate 145 bpm, and a controlled mechanical ventilation respiratory rate of 12/min. His temperature was unchanged. No breath sounds could be heard over the right lung field. Diminished breath sounds were audible over the left lung lobes. Rhonchi and crackles also could be heard over the left lung fields.

A chest x-ray taken earlier that morning by portable machine showed the left lung to be partially aerated with patches of atelectasis; the right lung was shown to be completely atelectatic. No pneumothorax was present. His hemodynamic status revealed an increased CVP, RAP, $\overline{PA}$, RVSWI, and PVR and a decreased PCWP, CO, SV, SVI, CI, LVSWI, and SVR.* His ABGs were as follows: pH 7.25, $PaCO_2$ 65 mm Hg, HCO_3^- 25 mmol/L, and PaO_2 54 mm Hg. The patient's oxygenation status showed an increased $\dot{Q}s/\dot{Q}t$, $C(a - \overline{v})O_2$, and O_2ER, and a decreased DO_2 and $S\overline{v}O_2$.† His SpO_2 was 86%.

---

*CVP, *Central venous pressure;* RAP, *right atrial pressure;* $\overline{PA}$, *mean pulmonary artery pressure;* RVSWI, *right ventricular stroke work index;* PVR, *pulmonary vascular resistance;* PCWP, *pulmonary capillary wedge pressure;* CO, *cardiac output;* SV, *stroke volume;* SVI, *stroke volume index;* CI, *cardiac index;* LVSWI, *left ventricular stroke work index;* SVR, *systemic vascular resistance.*

†$\dot{Q}s/\dot{Q}t$, *Cardiac output shunted/total cardiac output;* $C(a - \overline{v})O_2$, *arterial–mixed venous difference in oxygen content;* O_2ER, *oxygen extraction ratio;* DO_2, *total oxygen delivery;* $S\overline{v}O_2$, *mixed venous oxygen saturation.*

Response 2

Based on the previous information, write your SOAP in the following space.

S _____

_____

O _____

_____

_____

_____

_____

_____

Response 2–cont'd

A _____

P _____

72 HOURS AFTER ADMISSION

The patient's condition was classified as critical and unstable. His skin still appeared cyanotic, and his neck veins were severely distended. His vital signs were as follows: blood pressure 80/32, heart rate 190 bpm, controlled mechanical ventilation respiratory rate of 14/min, and rectal temperature 38.9° C (102° F). No breath sounds could be heard over the right lung fields. Diminished breath sounds were audible over the left lung. Rhonchi and crackles also could be heard over the left lung fields. Large amounts of yellow sputum were being suctioned from the patient's endotracheal tube.

A portable chest x-ray showed the left lung to be partially aerated, with patches of atelectasis more extensive than they had been 2 days before. The right lung was still shown to be airless. The radiologist also described early signs of adult respiratory distress syndrome (ARDS). No pneumothorax was present. The patient's electro-cardiogram demonstrated periodic premature ventricular contractions.

All the patient's hemodynamic values had worsened from earlier readings. His ABGs were as follows: pH 7.22, $Paco_2$ 71 mm Hg, HCO_3^- 24 mmol/L, and Pao_2 34 mm Hg. The man's oxygenation status had worsened progressively from readings made 2 days earlier; his Spo_2 was 61%. The patient's family was called, and the hospital priest was notified. He died 24 hours later.

Response 3

Based on the previous information, write your SOAP in the following space.

S _____

_____

O _____

_____

_____

_____

_____

_____

_____

_____

A _____

_____

_____

_____

_____

_____

_____

_____

Response 3–cont'd

P

Pneumothorax

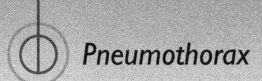

ADMITTING HISTORY

A 64-year-old white man is familiar to the respiratory care consult team. He has a history of chronic bronchitis and emphysema. Although he has not been hospitalized in more than 2 years, he received extensive care 4 years ago for a left lower lobe pneumonia that compromised his already severe chronic obstructive pulmonary disease (COPD). He was placed on the ventilator for 17 days. His medical record shows that hospital personnel experienced difficulty weaning him from the ventilator for both pathophysiologic and psychologic reasons. Despite this experience, he continues to smoke about 30 cigarettes a day, a habit he started when he joined the Navy at 19 years of age.

Since the episode 4 years ago, however, the man's medical history has been essentially unremarkable. As instructed, he schedules regular appointments with his doctor, twice a year. Most of the time he demonstrates a productive cough and wheezing. The man generally takes several medications, including daily dosages of antibiotics, xanthines, expectorants, and aerosolized sympathomimetics. Three or four times a week, for about 30 minutes, the man also performs a number of breathing exercises previously shown to him by the pulmonary rehabilitation team members.

He has worked as a janitor for more than 30 years in the local public school system. At the time of this admission he was 7 months from his retirement party. Even though he has suffered from chronic bronchitis and emphysema for many years, he has always been considered a reliable, hardworking employee by the school administration and his fellow workers. Although he often has gone to work feeling less than good, he always has been able to finish out the day without major problems. He seldom complains about his health so as not to draw attention to himself.

About 4 days before the present admission, however, he started to find it difficult to make it through the entire workday. He told his wife that he thought he was getting the flu, with symptoms of fatigue, chills, and a cough that was becoming worse and more productive. He nevertheless continued to go to work each day and made it to the end of the week. At home on Saturday, 2 hours before admission, he suddenly became very short of breath with minimal exertion. At one point he was unable to climb the stairs to his bedroom without stopping several times to rest. Concerned, his wife helped him into the car and drove him to the hospital.

PHYSICAL EXAMINATION

The man was in obvious respiratory distress. He was sitting in a wheelchair, with his arms anchored to the arms of the chair, using his accessory muscles of respiration. He was thin but well nourished. His skin appeared cyanotic, and his fingers were clubbed. He was pursed-lip breathing, and his chest was barrel shaped. He demonstrated a frequent, strong cough productive of large amounts of thick, yellow and green sputum. He stated that he had been coughing so much and so hard that his chest hurt around his left "collar bone."

His vital signs were as follows: blood pressure 145/85, heart rate 94 bpm, respiratory rate 20/min, and oral temperature 37.9° C (100.3° F). Palpation of the chest was unremarkable. Percussion revealed hyperresonant notes bilaterally. Auscultation revealed diminished breath sounds and rhonchi throughout both lung fields. His heart sounds were diminished. Expiration took him three times as long as inspiration.

His last pulmonary function test (PFT), taken about 6 months before at his last doctor's appointment, showed a moderate-to-severe obstructive disorder. His chest x-ray in the emergency room revealed dark, translucent lung fields, depressed and flattened hemidiaphragms, and a long, narrow heart. A small anterior pneumothorax (about 10%) also was noted between the second and third ribs on the left. His arterial blood gas values (ABGs) on room air were as follows: pH 7.53, $Paco_2$ 48 mm Hg, HCO_3^- 38 mmol/L, and Pao_2 57 mm Hg. His baseline ABGs at his last medical appointment were as follows: pH 7.42, $Paco_2$ 69 mm Hg, HCO_3^- 41 mmol/L, and Pao_2 74 mm Hg. The physician ordered guaifenesin (Robitussin), theophylline (Theo-Dur), bed rest with limited physical activity, and a respiratory care consult.

Response 1

Based on the previous information, write your SOAP in the following space.

S _____

_____

O _____

_____

_____

_____

_____

_____

_____

_____

_____

Response 1—cont'd

A _____

_____

_____

_____

_____

_____

_____

_____

P _____

_____

_____

_____

_____

3 HOURS LATER

The patient's primary nurse called a physician and paged respiratory care stat. A portable chest x-ray also was requested. The patient's respiratory distress had obviously worsened. The nurse stated that the patient had just pressed his bedside buzzer requesting help for his breathing. As the respiratory therapist walked into the patient's room, the man stated that he felt "like hell."

He appeared cyanotic and was pursed-lip breathing and perspiring. He demonstrated a frequent but weak cough, and when he did cough, he pulled his left arm to his side to brace himself. Although he expectorated only a small amount of sputum, he sounded "full." Rhonchi could be heard without the aid of a stethoscope. The sputum he did produce was still thick and yellow-green. His left anterior chest appeared hyperinflated and fixed, compared with the right.

His vital signs were as follows: blood pressure 95/55, heart rate 125 bpm and weak, and respiratory rate 28/min and shallow. Palpation of the chest was unremarkable. Percussion revealed hyperresonant notes bilaterally. Auscultation revealed diminished breath sounds and crackles, as well as rhonchi throughout the right lung. No breath sounds were audible over the left lung fields. Heart sounds could be heard to the right of the sternum. His ABGs were as follows: pH 7.24, $Paco_2$ 103 mm Hg, HCO_3^- 43 mmol/L, and Pao_2 37 mm Hg. His oxygen saturation measured by pulse oximetry (Spo_2) was 62%.

The chest x-ray showed that the patient's original small, left-sided pneumothorax had increased dramatically. The entire left lung now was collapsed; the left hemidiaphragm was significantly lower than the right; the mediastinum had shifted to the right, and patches of atelectasis were visible throughout the right lung.

The attending physician, along with a physician's assistant, inserted a chest tube in the left pleural cavity and began suction with negative pressure of -10 cm H_2O. The physician stated that in light of the problems the patient had experienced in the past, he did not want to commit the man to a ventilator. He requested respiratory care to assess the patient again, with a portable chest x-ray film to follow the first respiratory therapy treatments by 30 minutes.

Response 2

Based on the previous information, write your SOAP in the following space.

S _____

_____

O _____

_____

_____

_____

_____

_____

_____

_____

_____

_____

_____

A _____

_____

_____

Response 2–cont'd

P

30 MINUTES LATER

Although the patient was still in respiratory distress, his condition had improved. Tube suction had been increased. The chest x-ray showed that his left lung had re-expanded about 75%. The right lung fields were translucent, with no signs of atelectasis. The mediastinum had moved back to its normal position. The patient stated that he was feeling better. He still appeared cyanotic, was pursed-lip breathing, and was using his accessory muscles of respiration. Although he was still perspiring, the amount was less than it had been 30 minutes earlier.

No spontaneous cough or sputum production was observed. However, auscultation revealed diminished breath sounds and rhonchi over the right lung field. Breath sounds were diminished over the left lung area. His vital signs were as follows: blood pressure 145/85, heart rate 105 bpm, respiratory rate 22/min, and oral temperature 38° C (100.5° F). He was no longer cyanotic. Palpation of the chest was unremarkable. Percussion revealed hyperresonant notes bilaterally. Heart sounds no longer were heard over the right lung area. His ABGs were as follows: pH 7.35, $PaCO_2$ 85 mm Hg, HCO_3^- 41 mmol/L, and PaO_2 64 mm Hg. His SpO_2 was 90%.

Response 3

Based on the previous information, write your SOAP in the following space.

S _____

_____

O _____

_____

_____

_____

_____

_____

_____

A _____

_____

_____

_____

_____

_____

_____

P _____

_____

_____

_____

_____

PART VI

Disorders of the Pleura and Chest Wall

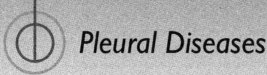

Pleural Diseases

15

ADMITTING HISTORY

Against her doctor's advice, a 38-year-old white woman discharged herself from the hospital about 2 months before the present admission. At that time she was admitted for severe right lower lobe pneumonia. After 5 days of treatment she became angry because she was not allowed to smoke. She was a longtime, three-pack-per-day smoker. When a nurse found her smoking in her hospital bed with a 2 L/min oxygen nasal cannula, the nurse quickly confiscated her cigarettes and matches.

The woman became upset. She told her doctor that this was the last straw and that she was going to leave the hospital on her own. Her doctor wanted her to remain so that a thorough follow-up could be performed for what was described as a "spot" on her lower right lung. The woman promised that she would make an appointment at the doctor's office the next week. She then got dressed and left. However, 2 days after she left the hospital she felt so much better that she decided the spot on her lung was not an issue for concern. The woman told her friends that smoking one pack of cigarettes made her feel better than 5 days' worth of nurses, doctors, and hospitals.

On the day of the present admission the woman appeared at the doctor's office without an appointment. She told the receptionist that something was very wrong. She thought that she had the flu and that it had been getting progressively worse over the last 4 days. At this time, she could speak in short sentences only and was unable to inhale deeply. Seeing that the woman was in obvious respiratory distress, the nurse interrupted the doctor. Within 5 minutes the doctor had the woman transported and admitted to the hospital a few blocks away.

PHYSICAL EXAMINATION

The woman appeared malnourished, exhibited poor personal hygiene, and had yellow tobacco stains around her fingers. She appeared to be in moderate-to-severe respiratory distress. Her skin was cyanotic, and her shirt was wet from perspiration. She demonstrated an occasional hacking, nonproductive cough. She stated that she could not take a deep breath and that maybe the problem stemmed from that spot on her lung.

Her vital signs were as follows: blood pressure 146/92, heart rate 112 bpm, and respiratory rate 36/min and shallow. She was slightly febrile, with an oral temperature of

37.7° C (99.8° F). Palpation showed that the trachea was shifted slightly to the left. Dull percussion notes were found over the right middle and right lower lobes. Auscultation revealed normal vesicular breath sounds over the left lung fields and upper right lobe. No breath sounds could be heard over the right middle and right lower lobes.

The patient's chest x-ray showed a large, right-sided pleural effusion. The right costophrenic angle demonstrated blunting, the right hemidiaphragm was depressed, and the right middle and lower lung lobes were partially collapsed and showed changes consistent with pneumonia (Fig. 15-1). The arterial blood gas values (ABGs) on a 3 L/min oxygen nasal cannula were as follows: pH 7.53, $Paco_2$ 24 mm Hg, HCO_3^- 19 mmol/L, and Pao_2 37 mm Hg. The oxygen saturation measured by pulse oximetry (Spo_2) was 44%. The doctor, assisted by the respiratory therapist, performed a thoracentesis on the patient at the bedside. Slightly more than 2 L of yellow fluid was withdrawn. The patient then was started on intravenous antibiotics. A portable chest x-ray was ordered, and a respiratory care consult was requested.

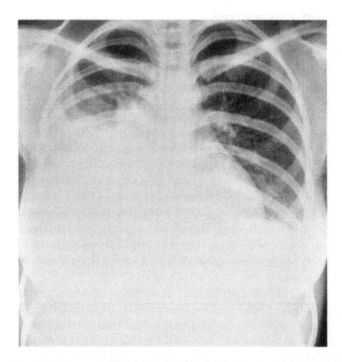

Fig. 15-1 Chest x-ray of a 38-year-old woman with pleural disease.

Response 1

Based on the previous information, write your SOAP in the following space.

S _____

_____

Response 1–cont'd

O _____

_____

_____

_____

_____

_____

_____

A _____

_____

_____

_____

_____

_____

_____

_____

_____

P _____

_____

_____

_____

_____

_____

_____

3 HOURS AFTER ADMISSION

At this time the patient was sitting up in bed and stated that although she was feeling better, she did not feel great. She still had an occasional dry-sounding, nonproductive cough. Her skin appeared pale and cyanotic. She was no longer perspiring, as she was when she was first admitted. Her vital signs were as follows: blood pressure 135/85, heart rate 100 bpm, respiratory rate 24/min, and temperature normal. Her respiratory efforts, however, no longer appeared shallow. Palpation was not remarkable. Dull percussion notes were found over the right middle and right lower lobes. Normal vesicular breath sounds were heard over the left lung and upper right lung. Loud bronchial breath sounds were audible over the right middle and right lower lobes.

The patient's chest x-ray showed a small, right-sided pleural effusion. Increased opacity was still present in the right middle and lower lung, consistent with pneumonia. The patient's trachea and mediastinum were in their normal positions. Her ABGs were as follows: pH 7.52, $Paco_2$ 29 mm Hg, HCO_3^- 22 mmol/L, and Pao_2 57 mm Hg. Her Spo_2 was 89%.

Response 2

Based on the previous information, write your SOAP in the following space.

S _____

_____

O _____

_____

_____

_____

_____

_____

_____

_____

A _____

_____

Response 2–cont'd

_____

_____

_____

_____

_____

_____

_____

_____

P _____

_____

_____

_____

_____

_____

_____

5 HOURS AFTER ADMISSION

Approximately 30 minutes before planning to call to update the physician, the respiratory care practitioner prepared a full SOAP. The patient was situated in a semi-Fowler's position. She appeared relaxed and alert. She stated that she had finally caught her breath. Although she still appeared pale, she did not look cyanotic. No spontaneous cough was observed at this time.

Her vital signs were as follows: blood pressure 128/79, heart rate 88 bpm, respiratory rate 16/min, and temperature normal. Palpation of the chest was unremarkable. Dull percussion notes were found over the right middle and right lower lobes. Normal vesicular breath sounds were heard over the left lung and right upper lobe. Bronchial breath sounds were audible over the right middle and right lower lobes. No current chest x-ray was available. The patient's ABGs were as follows: pH 7.45, $Paco_2$ 36 mm Hg, HCO_3^- 24 mmol/L, and Pao_2 77 mm Hg. Her Spo_2 was 92%.

Response 3

Based on the previous information, write your SOAP in the following space.

S _____

_____

O _____

_____

_____

_____

_____

_____

_____

A _____

_____

_____

_____

_____

_____

_____

P _____

_____

_____

_____

_____

_____

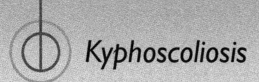

Kyphoscoliosis

16

ADMITTING HISTORY

A 62-year-old white woman began to develop kyphoscoliosis when she was 6 years old. She lived in the mountains of Virginia all her life, with her parents and later her two older sisters. Although she wore several different body braces until she was 17 years old, her disorder was classified as severe by the time she was 15 years old. The doctors, who were few and far between, always told her that she would have to learn to live with her condition the best she could, and as a general rule she did.

She finished high school with no other remarkable physical or personal problems. She was well liked by her classmates and was actively involved in the school newspaper and art club. After graduation she continued to live with her parents for a few more years. At 21 years of age she moved in with her two older sisters, who were buying a large farmhouse near a small but popular tourist town. All three sisters made various arts and crafts, which they sold at local tourist shops. The woman's physical disability and general health were relatively stable until she was about 40 years old. Around that time she started to experience frequent episodes of dyspnea, coughing, and sputum production. As the years progressed her baseline condition was marked by increasingly severe dyspnea.

Because the sisters rarely ventured into the city, the woman's medical resources were poor until she was introduced to a social worker at a nearby church. The church had just become part of an outreach program based in a large city nearby. The social worker was charmed by the woman and fascinated by the beauty of the colorful quilts she made.

The social worker, however, also was concerned by the woman's limited ability to move because of her severe chest deformity. In addition, the social worker thought that the woman's cough sounded serious. She noted that the woman appeared grayish-blue, weak, and ill. The sisters told the social worker that their sibling had had a bad cold for about 6 months. After much urging the social worker convinced the woman to travel, accompanied by her sisters, to the city to see a doctor at a large hospital associated with the church outreach program. On arrival the woman was admitted to the hospital. The sisters stayed in a nearby hotel room provided by the hospital.

PHYSICAL EXAMINATION

The woman appeared to be well nourished and suffering from severe kyphoscoliosis. The lateral curvature of the spine was twisted significantly to the patient's left. In addition, she also demonstrated anterior bending of the thoracic spine. She appeared older than her stated age, and she was in obvious respiratory distress. The patient stated that she was having trouble breathing. Her skin was cyanotic. She had digital clubbing, and her neck veins were distended, especially on the right side. The woman demonstrated a frequent but adequate cough. During each coughing episode she expectorated a moderate amount of thick, yellow sputum.

When the patient generated a strong cough, a large unilateral "bulge" appeared at the right anterolateral base of her neck, directly posterior to the clavicle. The patient referred to the bulge as her "Dizzy Gillespie" pouch. The doctor thought that the bulge was a result of the severe kyphoscoliosis, which had in turn stretched and weakened the suprapleural membrane that normally restricts and contains the parietal pleura at the apex of the lung. Because of the weakening of the suprapleural membrane, any time the woman produced a Valsalva's maneuver for any reason (e.g., for coughing), the increased intrapleural pressure herniated the suprapleural membrane outward. Despite the odd appearance of the bulge, the doctor did not consider it a serious concern at this time.

The patient's vital signs were as follows: blood pressure 160/100, heart rate 90 bpm, respiratory rate 18/min, and oral temperature 36.3° C (97.4° F). Palpation revealed a trachea deviated to the right. Dull percussion notes were produced over both lungs; crackles and rhonchi were heard over them as well. A pulmonary function test (PFT) conducted that morning showed vital capacity (VC), functional residual capacity (FRC), and residual volume (RV) between 45% and 50% of predicted values.

Although the patient's electrolytes were all normal, her hematocrit was 58%, and her hemoglobin level was 18 g/dl. A chest x-ray revealed a severe thoracic and spinous deformity, a mediastinal shift, an enlarged heart with prominent pulmonary artery segments bilaterally, and bilateral infiltrates in the lung bases consistent with pneumonia and atelectasis (Fig. 16-1). The patient's arterial blood gas values (ABGs)

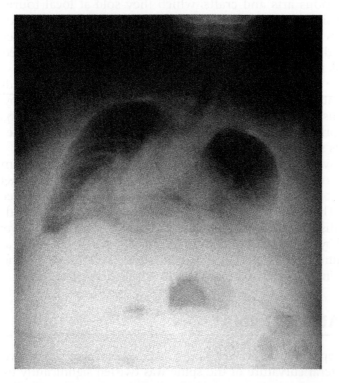

Fig. 16-1 Chest x-ray of a 62-year-old woman with kyphoscoliosis.

on room air were as follows: pH 7.52, $Paco_2$ 58 mm Hg, HCO_3^- 42 mmol/L, and Pao_2 49 mm Hg. Her oxygen saturation measured by pulse oximetry (Spo_2) was 78%. The physician requested a respiratory care consult and stated that mechanical ventilation was not an option at this time per the patient's request and his knowledge of the case.

Response 1

Based on the previous information, write your SOAP in the following space.

S _____

_____

O _____

_____

_____

_____

_____

_____

_____

_____

A _____

_____

_____

_____

_____

_____

_____

_____

Continued

Response 1—cont'd

P _____

_____

_____

_____

_____

_____

10 HOURS AFTER ADMISSION

The patient had not improved and was transferred to an intensive care unit. The physician had trouble titrating the cardiac drugs and decided to insert a pulmonary artery catheter, a central venous catheter, and an arterial line. Because of the woman's cardiac problems, several medical students, respiratory therapists, nurses, and doctors were constantly in and out of her room, performing and assisting in various procedures. As a result, working with the patient for any length of time was difficult, and the intensity of respiratory care was less than desirable. Eventually the patient's cardiac status stabilized, and the physician requested an update on the woman's pulmonary condition.

The respiratory therapist working on the pulmonary consult team found the patient in extreme respiratory distress. She was sitting up in bed, appeared frightened, and stated that she was extremely short of breath. Both of her sisters were in the room; one sister was putting cold towels on the patient's face while the other sister was holding the patient's hands. Both sisters were crying softly.

The woman's skin appeared cyanotic, and perspiration was visible on her face. Her neck veins were still distended. She demonstrated a weak, spontaneous cough. Although no sputum was noted, she sounded congested when she coughed. Dull percussion notes, crackles, and rhonchi were still present throughout both lungs. Her vital signs were as follows: blood pressure 180/120, heart rate 130 bpm, respiratory rate 26/min, and rectal temperature 37.8° C (100° F).

Several of the woman's hemodynamic indices were elevated: CVP, RAP, $\overline{PA}$, RVSWI, and PVR.* All other hemodynamic indices were normal. Her oxygenation indices were as follows: increased $\dot{Q}s/\dot{Q}T$ and O_2ER and decreased Do_2 and $S\bar{v}o_2$. Her $\dot{V}o_2$ and $C(a - \bar{v})o_2$ were normal.† No recent chest x-ray was available. Her ABGs were as follows: pH 7.57, $Paco_2$ 49 mm Hg, HCO_3^- 40 mmol/L, and Pao_2 43 mm Hg. Her Spo_2 was 76%.

---

*CVP, *Central venous pressure;* RAP, *right atrial pressure;* $\overline{PA}$, *mean pulmonary artery pressure;* RVSWI, *right ventricular stroke work index;* PVR, *pulmonary vascular resistance.*

†$\dot{Q}s/\dot{Q}T$, *Cardiac output shunted per total cardiac output;* O_2ER, *oxygen extraction ratio;* Do_2, *total oxygen delivery;* $S\bar{v}o_2$, *mixed venous oxygen saturation;* $\dot{V}o_2$, *oxygen consumption per unit time;* $C(a - \bar{v})o_2$, *arterial − mixed venous difference in oxygen content.*

Response 2

Based on the previous information, write your SOAP in the following space.

S _____

_____

O _____

_____

_____

_____

_____

_____

_____

A _____

_____

_____

_____

_____

_____

_____

_____

P _____

_____

_____

_____

_____

_____

24 HOURS AFTER ADMISSION

At this time the respiratory care practitioner found the patient watching the morning news on television with her two sisters. The woman was situated in a semi-Fowler's position eating the last few bites of her breakfast. The patient stated that she felt "so much better" and that "finally I have enough wind to eat some food."

Although her skin still appeared pale and cyanotic, she did not look as bad as she had the day before. On request she produced a strong cough and expectorated a small amount of white sputum. Her vital signs were as follows: blood pressure 140/85, heart rate 83 bpm, respiratory rate 14/min, and temperature normal. Chest assessment findings demonstrated crackles, rhonchi, and dull percussion notes over both lung fields. The rhonchi were less intense, however, than they had been the day before.

Although the patient's hemodynamic and oxygenation indices were better than they had been the day before, she still had room for improvement. Her hemodynamic parameters, still abnormal, revealed an elevated CVP, RAP, $\overline{PA}$, RVSWI, and PVR. All other hemodynamic indices were normal. Her oxygenation indices still showed an increased $\dot{Q}s/\dot{Q}t$ and O_2ER and a decreased DO_2 and $S\overline{v}O_2$. Her $\dot{V}O_2$ and $C(a - \overline{v})O_2$ were normal. The patient's chest x-ray taken earlier that morning showed some clearing of the pneumonia and atelectasis described on admission. Her ABGs were as follows: pH 7.45, $PaCO_2$ 73 mm Hg, HCO_3^- 48 mmol/L, and PaO_2 68 mm Hg. Her SpO_2 was 93%.

Response 3

Based on the previous information, write your SOAP in the following space.

S _____

_____

O _____

_____

_____

_____

_____

_____

_____

_____

Response 3–cont'd

A _____

_____

_____

_____

_____

_____

_____

_____

P _____

_____

_____

_____

_____

_____

_____

PART VII

Environmental Lung Diseases

Pneumoconiosis

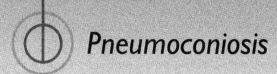

ADMITTING HISTORY

A 72-year-old man is well known to the treating hospital staff members, having received care there for more than 12 years. While in the U.S. Navy during World War II, he worked on the East Coast in the ship construction industry. After his discharge in 1945 he returned to his home in Mississippi for about 6 months; he then moved to Detroit, Michigan, and worked for an automobile manufacturer. His primary job for the next 20 years was undercoating automobiles.

In the early 1970s the man was transferred to a nearby automotive plant, where he worked on an assembly line, fastening bumpers and chrome trim to cars. He was well liked by his fellow workers and was considered a hard worker by the administration. When he retired in 1980, he was one of four supervisors in charge of the chrome trim assembly line.

Although the man smoked two packs a day for more than 40 years, his health was essentially unremarkable until about 4 years before he retired. At that time he started to experience periods of coughing, dyspnea, and weakness. A complete examination provided by the company concluded that the man had moderate pneumoconiosis.

Based on the man's work history the doctor speculated that the pneumoconiosis was caused by asbestos fibers. This speculation was confirmed later with a Perls' stain of sputum, and the diagnosis of asbestosis was noted in the patient's chart. Just before the man retired, his pulmonary function tests (PFTs) showed a mild-to-moderate combined restrictive and obstructive disorder.

Although the man was able to enjoy a couple of relatively good years of retirement with his wife, his health declined rapidly thereafter. His cough and dyspnea quickly became a daily problem. Despite his deteriorating health, the man continued to smoke. When he was 68 years old, he was hospitalized for 8 days to treat pneumonia and severe respiratory distress. When he was discharged at that time, his PFTs still showed a moderate-to-severe restrictive and obstructive disorder. He started using oxygen at home regularly.

Approximately 10 months before the current admission the man was hospitalized for congestive heart failure. He was treated aggressively and sent home within 5 days. At the time of discharge his PFT results showed that he had a severe restrictive and obstructive respiratory disorder. His arterial blood gas values (ABGs) on 2 L/min oxygen by nasal cannula were as follows: pH 7.38, $Paco_2$ 86 mm Hg, HCO_3^- 46 mmol/L, and Pao_2 63 mm Hg.

Approximately 3 hours before the current admission the man awoke from an afternoon nap extremely short of breath. His wife stated that he coughed almost continuously and that he had difficulty speaking. She measured his oral temperature, which read 38° C (100° F). Concerned, she drove her husband to the hospital emergency room.

PHYSICAL EXAMINATION

As the man was wheeled into the emergency room, he appeared nervous, weak, and in obvious respiratory distress. He was on a 1.5 L/min oxygen nasal cannula, which was connected to an E-tank that was attached to the wheelchair. His skin felt damp and clammy to the touch. He appeared pale and cyanotic. His neck veins were distended, and his fingers and toes were clubbed. He demonstrated a frequent but weak cough productive of a moderate amount of thick, whitish-yellow secretions. He had peripheral edema (3+) of the ankles and feet. He said this was the worst his breathing had ever been.

The patient's vital signs were as follows: blood pressure 180/96, heart rate 108 bpm, respiratory rate 32/min, and oral temperature 38.3° C (100.8° F). Palpation of the chest was negative. Percussion produced bilateral dull notes in the lung bases. Wheezing, rhonchi, and crackles were auscultated throughout both lungs. A pleural friction rub could be heard over the right middle lobe between the sixth and seventh ribs, between the anterior axillary line and midaxillary line.

The patient's lower lobes had a diffuse, "ground-glass" appearance on the chest x-ray. Irregularly shaped opacities in the right and left lower pleural spaces were identified by the radiologist as calcified pleural plaques. A possible infiltrate consistent with pneumonia also was visible in the right middle lobes. In addition, the chest x-ray suggested that the right side of the heart was moderately enlarged (Fig. 17-1). His ABGs on a 1.5 L/min oxygen nasal cannula were as follows: pH 7.56, $PaCO_2$ 51 mm Hg, HCO_3^- 38 mmol/L, and PaO_2 47 mm Hg.

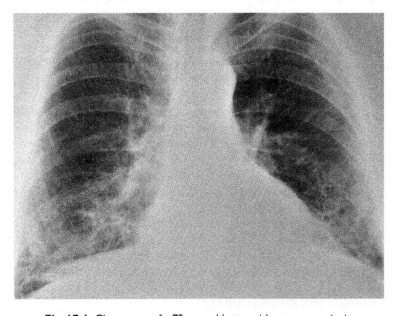

Fig. 17-1 Chest x-ray of a 72-year-old man with pneumoconiosis.

The physician started the patient on intravenous (IV) furosemide (Lasix) to treat the man's cor pulmonale and began administering an antibiotic to treat suspected pneumonia. Respiratory care was called to obtain a sputum culture, perform a respiratory care evaluation, and outline further respiratory therapy. The physician said that she did not want to commit the patient to a ventilator unless absolutely necessary.

Response 1

Based on the previous information, write your SOAP in the following space.

S _____

_____

O _____

_____

_____

_____

_____

_____

_____

_____

_____

A _____

_____

_____

_____

_____

_____

_____

_____

Response 1–cont'd

P _____

_____

_____

_____

_____

_____

THE NEXT MORNING

Throughout the night the patient's condition remained unstable. He continued to cough frequently but could not expectorate secretions very well on his own. When the therapist assisted the patient during coughing episodes, a moderate amount of thick, white and yellow sputum was produced. Even though he was conscious, alert, and able to follow simple directions, he did not answer any questions asked by the respiratory care practitioner regarding his breathing.

His skin was cold and damp to the touch, and he appeared short of breath. His color was improved, but he still appeared pale and cyanotic. His neck veins were still distended, although not so severely as they had been on admission, and edema of his ankles and feet could still be seen. The patient's vital signs were as follows: blood pressure 192/108, heart rate 113 bpm, respiratory rate 34/min, and oral temperature 38° C (100.4° F). Palpation of the chest was negative.

Dull percussion notes were elicited over the lung bases. Wheezing, rhonchi, and crackles continued to be auscultated throughout both lungs. A pleural friction rub could still be heard over the right middle lung between the sixth and seventh ribs, between the anterior axillary line and midaxillary line. No recent chest x-ray was available. His ABGs were as follows: pH 7.57, $Paco_2$ 47 mm Hg, HCO_3^- 36 mmol/L, and Pao_2 40 mm Hg. His oxygen saturation measured by pulse oximetry (Spo_2) was 77%.

Response 2

Based on the previous information, write your SOAP in the following space.

S _____

_____

Response 2–cont'd

O _____

_____

_____

_____

_____

_____

_____

_____

A _____

_____

_____

_____

_____

_____

_____

_____

_____

P _____

_____

_____

_____

_____

_____

_____

_____

20 HOURS LATER

At 6:15 AM the alarm on the patient's cardiac monitor sounded. The ECG strip showed several premature ventricular contractions followed by ventricular flutter and fibrillation. The head nurse called for a code blue. Cardiopulmonary resuscitation was started immediately. Because of the severe hypotension (blood pressure 80/50), epinephrine and dopamine were administered through the patient's IV line. Approximately 12 minutes into the code the patient exhibited a normal sinus rhythm. Spontaneous respiration were absent.

The patient was intubated, transferred to the intensive care unit (ICU), and placed on a mechanical ventilator. The initial ventilator settings were in assist control mode as follows: 12 breaths per minute, FIO_2 1.0, pressure support +4 cm H_2O, and +10 cm H_2O positive end-expiratory pressure (PEEP). His cardiopulmonary status remained unstable. Premature ventricular contractions were seen frequently on the ECG monitor. A pulmonary artery catheter and arterial line were inserted.

The patient's skin was pale, cyanotic, and clammy. His neck veins were still distended, and his ankles and feet were swollen. Vital signs were as follows: blood pressure 135/90, heart rate 84 bpm, and rectal temperature 38.3° C (100.8° F). Palpation of the chest wall was negative. Dull percussion notes were produced over the lung bases. Wheezing, rhonchi, and crackles continued to be auscultated throughout both lungs. Thick, greenish-yellow sputum was frequently suctioned from the patient's endotracheal tube.

A pleural friction rub still could be heard over the right middle lung lobe between the sixth and seventh ribs, between the anterior axillary line and midaxillary line. A chest x-ray had been taken but had not yet been interpreted by the radiologist. The patient's hemodynamic indices were as follows: elevated CVP, RAP, $\overline{PA}$, RVSWI, and PVR.* All other hemodynamic values were normal. His ABGs were as follows: pH 7.53, $Paco_2$ 56 mm Hg, HCO_3^- 38 mmol/L, and Pao_2 246 mm Hg. His Spo_2 was 98%.

---

*CVP, *Central venous pressure;* RAP, *right atrial pressure;* $\overline{PA}$, *mean pulmonary artery pressure;* RVSWI, *right ventricular stroke work index;* PVR, *pulmonary vascular resistance.*

Response 3

Based on the previous data, write your SOAP in the following space.

S _____

_____

O _____

_____

_____

Response 3–cont'd

_____

_____

_____

_____

_____

_____

A _____

_____

_____

_____

_____

_____

_____

P _____

_____

_____

_____

_____

_____

PART

PART VIII

Neoplastic Disease

Cancer of the Lungs

18

ADMITTING HISTORY

A 66-year-old retired man lives with his wife in a small, two-bedroom ranch house in Peoria, Illinois, during the summer months. During the rest of the year, they live in a 22-foot trailer in a retirement park just outside Las Vegas, Nevada. The trailer park is located conveniently on the casinos' shuttle bus route; a bus comes by at the top of every hour.

Both the man and his wife are described by their children as addicted gamblers. They gamble almost every day of the year. During the summer months they play keno and blackjack on the Par-A-Dice Riverboat Casino, which is docked along the shores of the Illinois River in downtown East Peoria. While in Las Vegas, they play bingo, blackjack, and the slot machines at several different casinos. They dress in matching warm-up suits, ride the bus to one of the casinos, and gamble until 10 or 11 PM every day.

Their children, adults with their own families, homes, and jobs in the Peoria area, are concerned about their parents' gambling. They have tried to no avail to get their parents to see a compulsive-gambling therapist, who actually is provided by the Par-A-Dice Riverboat Casino.

Their children's concern is justified. Their parents are always gambling on a shoe-string budget. Although they still own their trailer and small home in Peoria, within the last 2 years they have gambled away most of their life savings, which included stocks, bonds, and mutual funds. Because they let their health insurance premium lapse, their policy recently was canceled. They still receive a small monthly pension check, however, and some Social Security money.

Before he retired the man worked for 17 years as a boiler tender for Methodist Hospital in Peoria. He was also a part-time firefighter. For more than 52 years he smoked between two and a half and three packs of unfiltered cigarettes a day. While in Las Vegas about 3 months earlier the man began experiencing periods of dyspnea, coughing, and weakness. His cough was productive of small amounts of clear secretions. Also around this time his wife first noticed that his voice sounded hoarse.

Although he missed several days of gambling and remained in bed because of weakness, he did not seek medical attention. He hates doctors and thought that he suffered merely from a bad cold and the flu. When he returned to Peoria for the summer, however, the children became concerned and insisted that he see a doctor. Despite the man's lack of health insurance, two medical students from the University of Illinois, who were working as a team, ordered a full diagnostic workup.

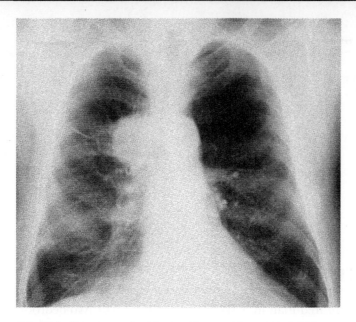

Fig. 18-1 Chest x-ray of a 66-year-old man with cancer of the lungs.

A pulmonary function test (PFT) showed that the man had a restrictive and obstructive pulmonary disorder. Computed tomography scanning revealed several masses, ranging from 2 to 5 cm in diameter, in the right and left mediastinum in the hilar regions. The masses, especially on the right side, also could be seen clearly on the posteroanterior chest radiograph (Fig. 18-1). Both the CT scan and the chest x-ray showed an increased opacity consistent with atelectasis of the medial basal segments of the left lower lobe as well.

A fiber-optic bronchoscopic examination was conducted by the pulmonary physician, with the assistance of a respiratory therapist trained in special procedures. It showed several large, protruding bronchial masses in the second- and third-generation bronchi of the right lung and the second-, third-, and fourth-generation bronchi of the left lung. During the bronchoscopy several mucus plugs were suctioned. Biopsy of three of the larger tumors was positive for squamous cell bronchogenic carcinoma, and the man was admitted to the hospital.

The physician told the patient that he had cancer and that his prognosis was poor. Treatment, at best, would be palliative. The patient asked what the odds were on his life expectancy. The physician stated that only about a 50% chance existed that he would live longer than 6 to 8 weeks. Surgery was out of the question. In the interim, however, the physician promised to do what was possible to make the man comfortable. The physician outlined a treatment plan of radiation therapy and chemotherapy and requested a respiratory care consult.

PHYSICAL EXAMINATION

The respiratory care practitioner reviewed the admitting history information in the patient's chart and found the man sitting up in bed in obvious respiratory distress. He appeared weak. His skin was cyanotic, and his face, arms, and chest were damp with perspiration. Wheezing could be heard with the aid of a stethoscope. He stated in a hoarse voice that he had coughed up a cup of sputum since breakfast 2 hours earlier. He demonstrated a weak cough every few minutes or so. His cough was productive of large amounts of blood-streaked sputum. The viscosity of the sputum was "thin." After each coughing episode he stated that he wanted a cigarette and then laughed.

His vital signs were as follows: blood pressure 155/85, heart rate 90 bpm, respiratory rate 22/min, and temperature normal. Palpation was unremarkable. Percussion produced dull notes over the left lower lobe. On auscultation, rhonchi, wheezing, and crackles could be heard throughout both lung fields. His arterial blood gas values (ABGs) on a 2 L/min oxygen nasal cannula were as follows: pH 7.51, $PaCO_2$ 29 mm Hg, HCO_3^- 22 mmol/L, and PaO_2 66 mm Hg. His oxygen saturation measured by pulse oximetry (SpO_2) was 92%.

Response 1

Based on the previous information, write your SOAP in the following space.

S _____

_____

O _____

_____

_____

_____

_____

_____

_____

_____

A _____

_____

_____

_____

_____

_____

Continued

Response 1–cont'd

P _____

3 DAYS AFTER ADMISSION

During morning rounds a respiratory care practitioner evaluated the patient. After reviewing the patient's chart, the practitioner went to the patient's bedside and discovered that the man was not tolerating the chemotherapy well. He had been vomiting off an on for the past 10 hours and was still in obvious respiratory distress. He appeared cyanotic and tired, and his hospital gown was wet from perspiration. His cough was still weak and productive of large amounts of moderately thick, clear and white sputum. He stated in a hoarse voice that he still was not breathing very well.

His vital signs were as follows: blood pressure 166/90, heart rate 95 bpm, respiratory rate 28/min, and temperature normal. Dull percussion notes were elicited over both the right and left lower lobes. Rhonchi, wheezing, and crackles were auscultated throughout both lung fields. His ABGs were as follows: pH 7.55, $PaCO_2$ 25 mm Hg, HCO_3^- 20 mmol/L, and PaO_2 53 mm Hg. His SpO_2 was 88%.

Response 2

Based on the previous information, write your SOAP in the following space.

S _____

Response 2–cont'd

O _____

_____

_____

_____

_____

_____

_____

_____

A _____

_____

_____

_____

_____

_____

_____

_____

_____

_____

P _____

_____

_____

_____

_____

_____

_____

_____

16 DAYS AFTER ADMISSION

Although the physician's original intention and hope was to discharge the patient soon, it was difficult to stabilize the man for any length of time. Over the past 2 weeks the patient had continued to be nauseated on a daily basis. He did, however, have occasional periods of relief in his ability to breathe, but he generally was in respiratory distress.

On this day the respiratory therapist observed and collected the following clinical data:

The patient was lying in bed in the supine position. His eyes were closed, and he was unresponsive to the therapist's questions.
The patient was in obvious respiratory distress. He appeared pale, cyanotic, and diaphoretic.
No cough was observed at this time, but rhonchi could easily be heard from across the patient's room. The nurse in the patient's room stated that the doctor had earlier called the rhonchi a "death rattle."

The patient's vital signs were as follows: blood pressure 170/105, heart rate 110 bpm, respiratory rate 11/min and shallow, and rectal temperature normal. Percussion was not performed. Rhonchi, wheezing, and crackles were heard throughout both lung fields. His ABGs were as follows: pH 7.28, $PaCO_2$ 63 mm Hg, HCO_3^- 27 mmol/L, and PaO_2 66 mm Hg. His SpO_2 was 90%.

Response 3

Based on the previous information, write your SOAP in the following space.

S _____

_____

O _____

_____

_____

_____

_____

_____

_____

_____

Response 3–cont'd

A _____

_____

_____

_____

_____

_____

_____

_____

P _____

_____

_____

_____

_____

_____

_____

PART IX

Diffuse Alveolar Diseases

Adult Respiratory Distress Syndrome

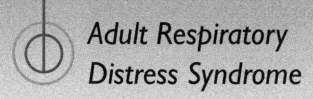

ADMITTING HISTORY

A 32-year-old man was involved in an automobile accident during an ice storm on the way to work. His car hit a patch of ice, spun out of control, and hit a cement bridge support. A 911 team spent 90 minutes extricating him from the car. He was stabilized at the accident site and then transported to the hospital. Although he was unconscious, he started to move and speak en route to the hospital. His speech was incoherent.

On admission he was hypotensive, conscious, and complaining of severe pain. When he was asked to identify specific pain sites, he stated that his whole body hurt. He had numerous facial lacerations and several broken teeth. A zygomatic arch was broken, and his right maxilla was fractured. He had a compound fracture of the left humerus, a Colles' fracture of the left radius, and several simple fractures of the first, second, and third phalanges on his left hand. A large bruise in the shape of a steering wheel could be observed easily over his anterior chest. He had a splintered fracture of his right tibia and fibula. Although the chest x-ray taken in the emergency room showed no rib fractures, bilateral patchy infiltrates could be seen throughout both lungs.

He was taken to surgery, where maxillofacial, plastic, and orthopedic surgeons worked to treat his multiple injuries. The patient was in the operating room for 16 hours. His surgery was described as successful, and the long-term prognosis was believed to be good. He was in the postoperative recovery room for 2 hours with no remarkable problems and then was transferred to the surgical intensive care unit (ICU).

On arrival in the ICU the man was breathing on his own, receiving supplemental oxygen via a 2 L/min nasal cannula. His general cardiopulmonary status was stable, and his recovery for the first 24 hours was as expected. At that time, however, the patient began to show signs of respiratory distress, and the attending physician ordered a respiratory care evaluation.

PHYSICAL EXAMINATION

The respiratory therapist assigned to assess and treat the patient gathered his clinical information. On inspection in the ICU the patient was in moderate respiratory distress. He appeared uncomfortable and complained that he could not move very well and that he was becoming short of breath. He stated that he had never been a smoker. His blood pressure was 125/78, heart rate was 93 bpm, respiratory rate was 21/min, and core temperature was normal. His skin appeared pale, and when he was asked to cough, he demonstrated an adequate, although nonproductive cough. On palpation, tenderness was noted over his anterior chest area bilaterally, and dull percussion notes were elicited over both lower lung regions. On auscultation, bilateral bronchial breath sounds were heard. His oxygen saturation measured by pulse oximetry (SpO_2) was 95%, and his arterial blood gas values (ABGs) on a 3 L/min oxygen nasal cannula were as follows: pH 7.51, $PaCO_2$ 29 mm Hg, HCO_3^- 22 mmol/L, and PaO_2 68 mm Hg. His chest x-ray showed "ground-glass" infiltrates throughout both lung fields (Fig. 19-1). The process was more extensive than that noted on admission.

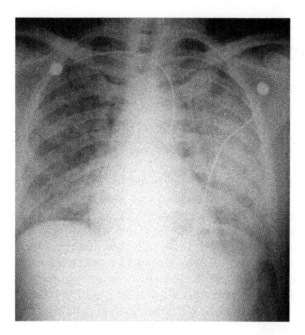

Fig. 19-1 Chest x-ray of a 32-year-old man with adult respiratory distress syndrome (ARDS).

Response 1

Based on the previous information, write your SOAP in the following space.

S _____

_____

O _____

_____

Response 1—cont'd

A

P

3 DAYS AFTER SURGERY

The patient paged the nurse and stated that he was feeling worse. Respiratory care was called. On observation the patient appeared cyanotic. His respiratory rate was 30/min, blood pressure was 165/95, heart rate was 110 bpm, and rectal temperature was 38.8° C (101.8° F). His cough was still nonproductive, and his anterior chest was still tender. Bronchial breath sounds and crackles were heard throughout both lung fields. His SpO_2 was 75%, and his ABGs were as follows: pH 7.56, $PaCO_2$ 24 mm Hg, HCO_3^- 18 mmol/L, and PaO_2 35 mm Hg. No recent chest x-ray was available, but one had been ordered.

Response 2

Based on the previous information, write your SOAP in the following space.

S _____

_____

O _____

_____

_____

_____

_____

_____

_____

A _____

_____

_____

_____

_____

_____

Response 2–cont'd

P _____

_____

_____

_____

_____

_____

_____

30 MINUTES LATER

The respiratory therapist assigned to monitor and evaluate the patient noted that the patient's respiratory rate was 18/min, blood pressure was 170/97, heart rate was 150 bpm, and rectal temperature was 37.8° C (100° F). He appeared cyanotic, and he no longer responded verbally when asked questions. On auscultation, bronchial breath sounds and crackles could be heard bilaterally. His SpO_2 was 69%, and his ABGs were as follows: pH 7.31, $PaCO_2$ 48 mm Hg, HCO_3^- 22 mmol/L, and PaO_2 31 mm Hg. A current chest x-ray showed increased opacities throughout both lung fields.

Response 3

Based on the previous information, write your SOAP in the following space.

S _____

_____

O _____

_____

_____

_____

Continued

Response 3–cont'd

A

P

KEY POINT QUESTIONS

For Adult Respiratory Distress Syndrome (DRG* 99/100)

1. Basic Concept Formation
   a. Which pulmonary conditions are associated with *trauma?*
   b. Which pulmonary conditions are associated with *infection?*
   c. Is adult respiratory distress syndrome (ARDS) an acute pulmonary illness usually requiring ventilator therapy?
2. Database Formation
   a. What are the predisposing and *etiologic factors* associated with ARDS?
   b. What is the systemic inflammatory response syndrome (SIRS)?
   c. What is your understanding of the *pathophysiology of ARDS?*
   d. What is your *vision of the pathologic process* of ARDS?
   e. What should be the *goals of therapy* for such patients?
   f. Which *standard therapist-driven protocols* would achieve these goals?
   g. List the *expected outcomes, possible adverse effects,* and *monitors* of each protocol you have selected.
3. Assessment
   a. Did this patient initially or subsequently demonstrate any *clinical manifestations* of ARDS? If so, what were they?
   b. Did this patient have any *risk factors* generally associated with SIRS or ARDS? If so, what were they?
   c. Did this patient demonstrate any of the *pathophysiologic alterations* associated with ARDS? If so, what were they?
   d. Which *specific clinical manifestations* did this patient demonstrate that helped you decide on the *severity* of his condition?
   e. Did the patient demonstrate any complications seen in other cases of ARDS?
4. Application
   a. Oxygen therapy (was/was not) indicated because _____ .
   b. Monitoring (was/was not) indicated because _____ .
   c. Hyperinflation therapy (was/was not) indicated because _____
   _____ .
5. Evaluation
   a. What are the expected *results* of each aspect of therapy selected?
   b. How should you *monitor* patient response?
   c. How can you increase or decrease the *intensity* or *frequency* of each modality as needed?
   d. What are the *advantages* and *disadvantages* of each treatment modality?
   e. What do you do if the patient improves?
   f. What do you do if he doesn't?
6. Boundary Awareness
   a. How would you know if *this* patient's condition does not improve or worsens?
   b. When should you ask a supervisor for help?
   c. When should you call the patient's physician?
   d. How would you recognize actual, impending, or worsening ventilatory failure in this patient?
   e. What *dangers* are present in the treatments you have selected?

DRG, Diagnosis-related group.

PART X

Chronic Noninfectious Parenchymal Diseases

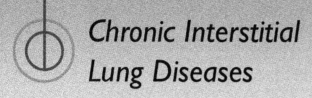

Chronic Interstitial Lung Diseases

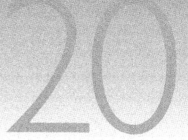

ADMITTING HISTORY

A 56-year-old black woman visited the health maintenance organization (HMO) clinic associated with her job because of shortness of breath and an ongoing dry, hacking cough. Before this visit she seldom saw a physician because she always perceived herself to be in perfect health. As a child, she was rarely ill and only saw her doctor for immunizations and preschool physicals.

The woman, a well-known editor at a prestigious publishing house, said that she had "little time" in her busy life to go through the "hassle" that her HMO required of her to make an appointment with a physician. Her last experience with the HMO system was frustrating. She especially did not approve of the physician assigned to see her.

On this day her worst fears were confirmed. For almost 5 hours she was shuffled from one waiting room to another, filling out forms, giving blood samples, and taking pulmonary function tests (PFT). During this visit the closest person to a physician she saw was a young physician's assistant (PA), who slowly took a thorough history. As the PA was closing her interview with the patient, the physician entered the room. The patient sarcastically stated, "You mean I'm finally going to see a real doctor?"

PHYSICAL EXAMINATION

On observation the patient appeared to be a stunning, well-nourished woman who looked much younger than her stated years. Her clothing was impeccable, and her jewelry was simple but elegant. The woman stated that she had made an appointment because of her recent inability to participate in aerobic exercise classes at work. She said that her shortness of breath, which had worsened progressively over the past several weeks, was accompanied by a dry, hacking cough. She said that her cough was especially annoying. It awakened her from sleep at night. At first, she said, she had tried to cut down on her aerobics classes, but recently she had been unable to tolerate them at all. She said that she had never smoked.

As she talked, the woman frequently demonstrated pursed-lip breathing. Her cough was frequent, dry, and nonproductive and was obviously annoying to her. She demonstrated a mild-to-moderate degree of digital clubbing, and her nail beds were cyanotic. She also demonstrated a mild degree of peripheral edema, and her neck veins were slightly distended. Her liver was enlarged and tender.

The woman's vital signs were as follows: blood pressure 145/90, heart rate 96 bpm, respiratory rate 28/min, and temperature normal. On auscultation, bronchial breath sounds and crackles could be heard bilaterally. Over the lung bases, tactile and vocal fremitus were notable. Rare wheezes were heard intermittently. Percussion was unremarkable.

Her PFT findings obtained a few hours earlier showed both a restrictive and an obstructive lung disorder, and the pulmonary carbon monoxide diffusion capacity (D_{LCO}) was 50% of the value predicted. Her chest x-ray revealed bilateral diffuse interstitial infiltrates and nodular densities in her lower lung lobes. Air bronchograms also were visible. Her heart was enlarged, suggesting right ventricular hypertrophy (Fig. 20-1). Her laboratory work showed an increase in immunoglobulin M (IgM), immunoglobulin G (IgG), and immunoglobulin A (IgA) antibodies. Her arterial blood gas values (ABGs) on room air were as follows: pH 7.53, Pa_{CO_2} 29 mm Hg, HCO_3^- 21 mmol/L, and Pa_{O_2} 61 mm Hg. At this point the physician elected to admit the woman to the hospital. The physician also requested a respiratory care consultation and scheduled a transbronchial lung biopsy.

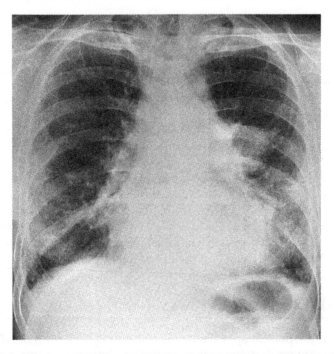

Fig. 20-1 Chest x-ray of a 56-year-old woman with chronic interstitial lung disease.

Response 1

Based on the previous information, write your SOAP in the following space.

S _____

_____

Response 1 – cont'd

O

A

P

2 DAYS AFTER ADMISSION

The respiratory care practitioner found the patient sitting up in bed editing a manuscript. She complained to the therapist that she had a lot of work to do and that she was getting tired of being in the hospital. Despite her verbal enthusiasm to leave, she appeared weak, fatigued, and in obvious respiratory distress. She still had a frequent, dry cough. She often demonstrated pursed-lip breathing as she talked, and her nail beds were still cyanotic.

Her vital signs were as follows: blood pressure 142/91, heart rate 90 bpm, respiratory rate 23/min, and temperature normal. On auscultation, bronchial breath sounds and crackles were audible bilaterally. The histology report regarding the transbronchial lung biopsy established a diagnosis of sarcoidosis, after which she was started on oral corticosteroids (Prednisone, 40 mg/day).

A morning chest x-ray showed unchanged bilateral diffuse interstitial infiltrates and nodular densities in the lower lung lobes. Air bronchograms also were visible. A gallium lung scan indicated moderate pulmonary activity. Evidence of cor pulmonale was still present. The patient's peak expiratory flow rate (PEFR) both before and after bronchodilator therapy was 280 L/min. Her ABGs were as follows: pH 7.48, $PaCO_2$ 32 mm Hg, HCO_3^- 23 mmol/L, and PaO_2 67 mm Hg. The woman's oxygen saturation measured by pulse oximetry (SpO_2) was 94%.

Response 2

Based on the previous information, write your SOAP in the following space.

S _____

_____

O _____

_____

_____

_____

_____

_____

_____

_____

_____

Response 2—cont'd

A _____

_____

_____

_____

_____

_____

_____

_____

_____

_____

P _____

_____

_____

_____

_____

_____

_____

_____

3 DAYS LATER

The physician requested a repeat respiratory care evaluation and recommendations regarding the patient's discharge. The respiratory care practitioner noted that the patient was not in as much respiratory distress on her present oxygen setting. Although she appeared comfortable, she still had a frequent dry, hacking cough and demonstrated pursed-lip breathing as she talked. She stated that she felt much better. Her nail beds no longer appeared cyanotic.

Her vital signs were as follows: blood pressure 133/86, heart rate 86 bpm, respiratory rate 15/min, and temperature normal. On auscultation, bronchial breath sounds were heard bilaterally. A morning chest x-ray showed no change in the bilateral diffuse interstitial infiltrates and nodular densities. Air bronchograms again were seen. Her ABGs on supplemental oxygen at 3 L/min per nasal cannula were as follows: pH 7.44, $PaCO_2$ 36 mm Hg, HCO_3^- 23 mmol/L, and PaO_2 84 mm Hg. The patient's SpO_2 was 95%.

Response 3

Based on the previous information, write your SOAP in the following space.

S _____

_____

O _____

_____

_____

_____

_____

_____

_____

A _____

_____

_____

_____

_____

_____

_____

P _____

_____

_____

_____

_____

_____

PART XI

Neurologic Disorders and Sleep Apnea

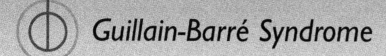

Guillain-Barré Syndrome

ADMITTING HISTORY/PHYSICAL EXAMINATION

A 48-year-old career U.S. Navy physician visited the hospital base clinic because of the acute onset of severe muscle weakness. He joined the Navy immediately after medical school. Throughout his time in the service he had the opportunity to pursue his passion—competitive water ski jumping. For many years he was the first-place winner at most tournaments, including the nationals held yearly. For almost 25 years he progressed through the age divisions, always remaining the top seed, always capturing the highest title.

The man was in outstanding physical condition. He was an avid runner and weight lifter, and during the off season he often traveled to a warm climate to practice his water ski jumping. He never smoked and was never hospitalized. He had an occasional cold, for which he was treated by his peers. About 2 years ago he began to focus all his attention on his 19-year-old son, who was quickly following in his footsteps, having just captured the Men's 1 division himself.

The man stated that he had felt good until 2 weeks before his admission, at which time he experienced a flulike syndrome for 3 days. About 10 days after returning to work, he noticed a tingling sensation in his feet during his morning patient rounds. By dinner time that same day the tingling sensation had radiated from his feet to about the level of his knees. Thinking that he was tired from being on his feet all day, he went to bed early that evening. The next morning, however, his legs were completely numb, although he could still move them. Becoming alarmed, he asked his son to drive him to the clinic. After examining him, his doctor (a personal friend) admitted him for a diagnostic workup and observation.

Over the next 3 days the laboratory results showed that the patient's cerebrospinal fluid had an elevated protein concentration with a normal cell count. The electrodiagnostic studies showed a progressive ascending paralysis of the man's arms and legs. He began to have difficulty eating and swallowing his food. The respiratory care practitioners, who were monitoring his vital capacity, pulse oximetry, and arterial blood gas values (ABGs), reported a progressive deterioration in all the values. A diagnosis of Guillain-Barré syndrome was placed in the patient's chart.

When the man's ABGs reached pH 7.31, $Paco_2$ 49 mm Hg, HCO_3^- 24 mmol/L, and Pao_2 86 mm Hg (on a 2 L/min oxygen nasal cannula), the respiratory therapist called the doctor and reported the assessment of acute ventilatory failure. The doctor transferred the patient to the intensive care unit (ICU), intubated him, and placed him on a mechanical ventilator. The initial ventilator settings were as follows: intermittent mechanical ventilation (IMV) mode, 12 breaths per minute, tidal volume 0.85 L, and F_{IO_2} 0.40.

Approximately 15 minutes after the patient was committed to the ventilator, he appeared comfortable. No spontaneous breaths were noted between the 12 intermittent mandatory ventilations. His vital signs were as follows: blood pressure 126/82 and heart rate 68 bpm. He was afebrile. A portable chest x-ray revealed that the endotracheal tube was in a good position and the lungs were adequately aerated. Normal vesicular breath sounds were auscultated over both lung fields. His ABGs were as follows: pH 7.51, Pa_{CO_2} 29 mm Hg, HCO_3^- 22 mmol/L, and Pa_{O_2} 204 mm Hg. His oxygen saturation measured by pulse oximetry (Sp_{O_2}) was 98%.

Response 1

Based on the previous information, write your SOAP in the following space.

S _____

_____

O _____

_____

_____

_____

_____

_____

_____

A _____

_____

_____

_____

_____

_____

_____

Response 1–cont'd

P _____

_____

_____

_____

_____

_____

3 DAYS AFTER ADMISSION

The patient's cardiopulmonary status so far had been unremarkable. No improvement was seen in his muscular paralysis. No changes had been made in his ventilator settings over the past 48 hours. His skin color appeared good. Palpation and percussion of the chest were unremarkable. On auscultation, however, crackles and rhonchi could be heard over both lung fields.

Moderate amounts of thick, white, clear secretions were being suctioned from the patient's endotracheal tube regularly. His vital signs were as follows: blood pressure 124/83, heart rate 74 bpm, and rectal temperature 37.7° C (99.8° F). A recent portable chest x-ray revealed no significant pathologic process. His ABGs were as follows: pH 7.44, $PaCO_2$ 35 mm Hg, HCO_3^- 24 mmol/L, and PaO_2 98 mm Hg. His SpO_2 was 97%.

Response 2

Based on the previous information, write your SOAP in the following space.

S _____

_____

O _____

_____

_____

_____

Continued

Response 2–cont'd

A

P

5 DAYS AFTER ADMISSION

The patient's muscular paralysis remained unchanged. His skin color appeared good, and no remarkable information was noted during palpation and percussion. Although crackles and rhonchi could still be heard over both lung fields, they were not as intense as they had been 48 hours earlier. A small amount of clear secretions was suctioned from the patient's endotracheal tube. His vital signs were as follows: blood pressure 118/79, heart rate 68 bpm, and temperature normal. A recent portable chest x-ray appeared normal. His ABGs were as follows: pH 7.42, $PaCO_2$ 37 mm Hg, HCO_3^- 24 mmol/L, and PaO_2 97 mm Hg. His SpO_2 was 97%. The sputum culture was unremarkable.

Response 3

Based on the previous information, write your SOAP in the following space.

S _____

_____

O _____

_____

_____

_____

_____

_____

_____

_____

A _____

_____

_____

_____

_____

_____

_____

P _____

_____

_____

_____

_____

_____

Based on the previous information, write out SOAP in the following space.

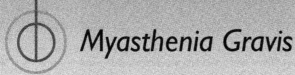

Myasthenia Gravis

ADMITTING HISTORY

A 35-year-old Spanish-American woman is a schoolteacher with a 3-year-old son and an unemployed husband who is still "finding his real place in life." The woman is a high achiever. Recently she received her doctoral degree in education but has continued to work in the classroom with the grade-school children she loves so much. She was named Teacher of the Year in the large city where she lives. Her colleagues at school consider her a nonstop worker. She has never smoked.

At home she is always on the move. She has just finished remodeling her kitchen and two bathrooms. She also does her own backyard landscaping on the weekends, a job she particularly enjoys. She reads and plays with her son whenever they have time together. Although she enjoys cooking (a skill she learned from her mother), she does not like to grocery shop. Fortunately this is a chore that her husband enjoys.

Three weeks before the current admission the woman noticed that her eyes "felt tired." She began to experience slight double vision. Thinking that she was working too hard, she slowed down a bit and went to bed earlier for about a week. However, she progressively felt weaker. Her legs quickly became tired, and she began having trouble chewing her food. Concerned, the woman finally went to see her doctor. After reviewing the woman's recent history and performing a careful physical examination, the physician admitted her to the hospital for further evaluation and treatment.

Over the next 48 hours the woman's physical status declined progressively. After the administration of edrophonium (Tensilon), her muscle strength increased significantly for about 10 minutes. Electromyography disclosed extensive muscle involvement and a high degree of fatigability in all the affected muscles. A diagnosis of myasthenia gravis was noted in the patient's chart.

The woman began to choke and aspirate food during meals, and a nasogastric feeding tube was inserted. Her speech became more and more slurred. Her upper eyelids drooped, and she was unable to hold her head off her pillow on request. The respiratory therapists who monitored her vital capacity, pulse oximetry, and arterial blood gas values (ABGs) reported a progressive worsening in all parameters.

When the woman's ABGs were pH 7.35, $PaCO_2$ 45 mm Hg, HCO_3^- 24 mmol/L, and PaO_2 69 mm Hg (on room air), the respiratory therapist called the physician and reported an assessment of impending ventilatory failure. The doctor had the patient transferred to the intensive care unit, intubated, and placed on a mechanical ventilator. The initial ventilator settings were as follows: intermittent mechanical ventilation (IMV) mode, 10 breaths per minute, tidal volume 0.8 L, and FIO_2 0.5.

Approximately 25 minutes after the patient was placed on the ventilator, she appeared stable. No spontaneous ventilations were seen. Her vital signs were as follows: blood pressure 132/86, heart rate 90 bpm, and rectal temperature 38° C (100.5° F). A portable chest x-ray had been ordered but not yet taken. Normal vesicular breath sounds were auscultated over the right lung, and diminished-to-absent breath sounds were auscultated over the left lung. On an FIO_2 of 0.5, her ABGs were as follows: pH 7.28, $PaCO_2$ 58 mm Hg, HCO_3^- 24 mmol/L, and PaO_2 52 mm Hg. Her oxygen saturation measured by pulse oximetry (SpO_2) was 80%.

Response 1

Based on the previous information, write your SOAP in the following space.

S _____

_____

O _____

_____

_____

_____

_____

_____

_____

A _____

_____

_____

_____

_____

_____

_____

Response 1–cont'd

P _____

_____

_____

_____

_____

_____

45 MINUTES LATER

After the patient's endotracheal tube was pulled back 4 cm, normal vesicular breath sounds could be auscultated over both lungs. The chest x-ray confirmed that the endotracheal tube was in a good position above the carina and that both lungs were adequately aerated.

Her vital signs were as follows: blood pressure 123/75, heart rate 74 bpm, and temperature normal. The ventilator settings were readjusted, and repeat ABGs were as follows: pH 7.53, $PaCO_2$ 27 mm Hg, HCO_3^- 22 mmol/L, and PaO_2 176 mm Hg. Her SpO_2 was 98%.

Response 2

Based on the previous information, write your SOAP in the following space.

S _____

_____

O _____

_____

_____

_____

_____

Continued

Response 2—cont'd

A _____

P _____

3 DAYS AFTER ADMISSION

No changes had needed to be made in the patient's ventilator settings over the previous 48 hours. No improvement was seen in her muscular paralysis. The woman appeared pale, and her vital signs were as follows: blood pressure 146/88, heart rate 92 bpm, and temperature 37.9° C (100.2° F). Large amounts of thick, yellowish sputum were being suctioned from her endotracheal tube approximately every 30 minutes.

Rhonchi were auscultated over both lung fields. A sputum sample was obtained and sent to the laboratory to be cultured. A recent portable chest x-ray showed a new infiltrate in the right lower lobe consistent with pneumonia or atelectasis. The ABGs were as follows: pH 7.28, $Paco_2$ 36 mm Hg, HCO_3^- 17 mmol/L, and Pao_2 41 mm Hg. Her Spo_2 was 69%.

Response 3

Based on the previous information, write your SOAP in the following space.

S _____

_____

O _____

_____

_____

_____

_____

_____

_____

_____

A _____

_____

_____

_____

_____

_____

_____

_____

_____

Continued

Response 3–cont'd

P

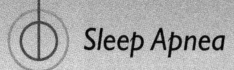

Sleep Apnea

ADMITTING HISTORY

A 55-year-old white man had been in the U.S. Marine Corps for more than 25 years when he retired with honors at 46 years of age with the rank of sergeant. He did tours in Vietnam, Grenada, and Beirut. His last assignment was in Iraq and Kuwait during Operation Desert Storm. During his military career he received several medals, including a Purple Heart for a leg wound received in Vietnam while he pulled a fellow marine to safety. During his last 3 years in the service he was assigned to a desk job, working with new recruits as they progressed through various stages of boot camp.

Although it was not mandatory that he retire, he felt that it was time. He had gained a great deal of weight over the years, and his ability to meet the physical challenge of being a marine had become progressively more difficult. In addition, when he was doing paper work at his office, he was aware that he was catnapping while on the job. He knew that if he had observed a fellow marine doing the same, he would have been quick to issue a severe reprimand. In view of these developments the man regretfully retired from the service.

For a few years after he retired he continued to work for the Marines as a volunteer at a local recruitment office. At first he enjoyed this job a great deal. He often found that his military experiences enhanced his ability to talk to new recruits. Over the past few years, however, he had found it progressively more difficult to work. His attendance had become increasingly sporadic. He was often tardy for work. He told the other recruitment volunteers that he was always tired and was experiencing severe morning headaches. His co-workers frequently found him irritable and quick to anger.

The man was having trouble at home too. Several months before this admission his wife had started sleeping in a room vacated by their daughter, who had recently married. She said that she no longer could sleep with her husband because of his loud snoring and constant thrashing in bed. About this time the man became clinically depressed and sexually impotent. Despite much discussion and encouragement from his wife, he did not seek medical advice until he became extremely short of breath a few hours before this admission. His wife drove him to the local emergency room, where he was evaluated.

PHYSICAL EXAMINATION

On observation the man appeared to be in severe respiratory distress. He was obese, weighing more than 160 kg (355 lb), and perspiring profusely. His skin appeared cyanotic, and his neck veins were distended. He had edema (4+) of his feet and legs extending to midcalf. His blood pressure was 194/118, heart rate was 78 bpm, respiratory rate was 22/min, and temperature was normal. Although the man was in obvious discomfort, he stated that he was breathing OK. His wife quickly piped up, "There's that damn marine coming out again."

The man's breath sounds were normal but diminished. The diminished breath sounds were believed to be due primarily to the patient's obesity. Palpation was unremarkable, and percussion was unreliable because of the obesity. A chest x-ray showed cardiomegaly; the lungs appeared normal. To treat presumed cor pulmonale the physician immediately started the patient on diuretics. His arterial blood gas values (ABGs) on room air were as follows: pH 7.54, $Paco_2$ 58 mm Hg, HCO_3^- 48 mmol/L, and Pao_2 52 mm Hg. His oxygen saturation measured by pulse oximetry (Spo_2) was 87%.

Because of the patient's history and present clinical manifestations, the respiratory therapist on duty suspected that the man suffered from obstructive sleep apnea. The therapist suggested this to the emergency room physician, who requested a polysomnographic study. The physician agreed and asked the respiratory therapist to document her assessment.

Response 1

Based on the previous information, write your SOAP in the following space.

S _____

_____

O _____

_____

_____

_____

_____

_____

_____

Response 1–cont'd

A _____

_____

_____

_____

_____

_____

_____

_____

P _____

_____

_____

_____

_____

_____

OVER THE NEXT 72 HOURS

The diagnosis of severe obstructive sleep apnea was quickly established. Along with the patient's classic history of obstructive sleep apnea, the polysomnogram documented more than 325 periods of obstructive apnea. The continuous positive airway pressure (CPAP) titration study indicated that 12 cm H_2O CPAP was required to treat the apneic syndrome. In addition to the patient's short, muscular neck and extreme obesity, an oropharyngeal examination revealed a small mouth and large tongue for his body size. The free margin of the soft palate hung low in the oropharynx, nearly obliterating the view behind it. The uvula was widened (4+) and elongated; the tonsillar pillars were widened (3+). Air entry through the nares was reduced bilaterally. A laboratory report showed the patient's hemocrit to be 51% and hemoglobin level to be 17 g/dl.

A complete pulmonary function test (PFT) showed that the man had a severe restrictive disorder. In addition, a saw-toothed pattern was seen in the maximal inspiratory and expiratory flow-volume loops. A chest x-ray obtained on the patient's second day of hospitalization showed reduction in heart size, and the lung parenchyma were clear. A brisk diuresis was in process. The patient stated that he was breathing much better.

On inspection the patient no longer appeared short of breath. Although he still appeared flushed, he did not look as cyanotic as he had on admission. His neck veins were no longer distended, and the peripheral edema of his legs and feet had improved. His breath sounds were clear but diminished. His room air ABGs were as follows: pH 7.38, Pa_{CO_2} 82 mm Hg, HCO_3^- 44 mmol/L, and Pa_{O_2} 66 mm Hg. His Sp_{O_2} was 91%. The physician again called for a respiratory care evaluation.

Response 2

Based on the previous information, write your SOAP in the following space.

S _____

_____

O _____

_____

_____

_____

_____

_____

_____

_____

A _____

_____

_____

_____

_____

_____

_____

Response 2–cont'd

P

PART XII

Newborn and Early Childhood Respiratory Disorders

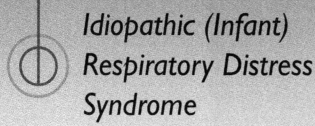

Idiopathic (Infant) Respiratory Distress Syndrome

ADMITTING HISTORY

A 1644 g (3 lb, 10 oz) boy was born 8 weeks early (at 32 weeks' gestation). The nurses were concerned about the mother's lack of interest in her baby's care. The mother is an unmarried, 17-year-old white high school dropout who plans to put the child up for adoption. Before this admission the mother, whose pregnancy was considered high risk, was seen for prenatal care only once. At the prenatal visit she was accompanied by her sister, who lived with her. Shortly after this visit the sister moved to a large nearby town, where she planned to become a certified nurse's assistant. The mother continued to live in their mobile home with her boyfriend, who was out of work. She is a checkout clerk at a small grocery store.

After the baby's birth the mother appeared moderately nervous as she sat up in bed talking to the social worker in preparation for her discharge. She appeared thin and poorly nourished and constantly requested to go to the smoking room. Because of the mother's obvious disinterest, little progress was made regarding her follow-up, the baby's present condition, or the adoption. Despite having given birth only 5 hours previously, she appeared quite anxious to be discharged.

PHYSICAL EXAMINATION

In the neonatal intensive care unit the baby appeared to be in mild respiratory distress. His Apgar scores at delivery were 4 and 6. On observation the baby appeared mildly cyanotic and demonstrated intercostal retractions and nasal flaring with all respirations. A mild, gruntlike cry was noted.

The baby's vital signs were as follows: blood pressure 50/20, apical heart rate 180 bpm, respiratory rate 74/min, and rectal temperature 37.1° C (98.8° F). Auscultation revealed bilateral crackles and sighing breath sounds. A stat chest x-ray (Fig. 24-1) showed mild haziness and air bronchograms in both lung bases consistent with the onset of infant respiratory distress syndrome (IRDS). The infant was placed on an FIO_2 of 0.4 via an oxygen hood. Umbilical arterial blood gas values (ABGs) were as follows: pH 7.52, $PaCO_2$ 29 mm Hg, HCO_3^- 21 mmol/L, and PaO_2 49 mm Hg.

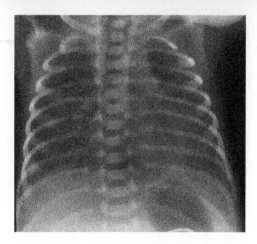

Fig. 24-1 Chest x-ray of an 8-week-premature newborn boy with idiopathic infant respiratory distress syndrome.

Response 1

Based on the previous information, write your SOAP in the following space.

S

O

A

Response 1–cont'd

P _____

16 HOURS AFTER DELIVERY

At this time the baby was placed on a time-cycled, pressure-limited synchronized intermittent mandatory ventilation (SIMV) rate of 30/min, inspiratory time of 0.5 seconds, peak inspiratory pressure (PIP) of 20 cm H_2O, FIO_2 of 0.6, and positive end-expiratory pressure (PEEP) of 3 cm H_2O. The baby had no spontaneous breaths. His blood pressure was 60/40, and the apical heart rate was 184 bpm. On auscultation, harsh bronchial breath sounds and fine crackles could be heard bilaterally. A recent chest x-ray revealed a dense, "ground-glass" appearance throughout both lung fields. Umbilical ABGs were as follows: pH 7.28, $PaCO_2$ 53 mm Hg, HCO_3^- 19 mmol/L, and PaO_2 57 mm Hg.

Response 2

Based on the previous information, write your SOAP in the following space.

S _____

Continued

Response 2—cont'd

O

A

P

48 HOURS LATER

The baby remained intubated and on mechanical ventilation. The ventilator was in the continuous positive airway pressure (CPAP) mode at a pressure setting of 3 cm H_2O, with an FIO_2 of 0.45. The infant's vital signs showed a blood pressure of 74/50, an apical heart rate of 120 bpm, a spontaneous respiratory rate of 42/min, and a normal temperature. On auscultation, clear, normal vesicular breath sounds were heard. A morning chest x-ray revealed substantial improvement in the lung fields. Umbilical ABGs were as follows: pH 7.42, $PaCO_2$ 37 mm Hg, HCO_3^- 24 mmol/L, and PaO_2 162 mm Hg.

Response 3

Based on the previous information, write your SOAP in the following space.

S _____

_____

O _____

_____

_____

_____

_____

_____

_____

_____

A _____

_____

_____

_____

_____

_____

_____

Continued

Response 3–cont'd

P

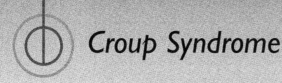

Croup Syndrome

ADMITTING HISTORY

Approximately 3 days before Christmas a 3-year-old boy appeared to be a typical, healthy child. He was energetic and curious, and his attention span was short. He generally played well with other children, and at his day-care center he was well liked and considered a happy child by the staff members. On this day, however, he often became frustrated and angry, and at one point a staff member had to stop a fight between the boy and a girl. The staff member noted that the boy's face appeared flushed and felt warm to the touch. Because the flu was going around, she thought that the boy could be coming down with it. At this point the boy's mother was called.

At home the mother checked her son's temperature, which was normal. Because he felt warm, however, she gave him liquid acetaminophen (Tylenol). For lunch the boy ate about three bites of a peanut butter sandwich and some grapes and drank about half a glass of juice. Although his mother wanted him to take a nap, he insisted that he was not tired. The boy then began to play with his father's Lionel train underneath the Christmas tree. Approximately 10 minutes later the boy was asleep while the train was still running. His mother then placed him in his bed.

Although the boy slept through the night, he was lethargic the next morning and frequently complained to his mother that he did not feel good. Even though the boy's temperature was normal, his mother gave him more liquid acetaminophen. For breakfast he ate a few bites of cereal and had some juice. He then wrapped himself in a blanket in front of the television set, coughing occasionally. By noon the mother noticed that her son's cough was more frequent and had developed a barking quality. She also noted that his voice sounded hoarse. By late afternoon the boy's condition has worsened progressively, and he told his mother he was having trouble breathing. Becoming worried, the mother carried him to the car and drove him to the hospital emergency room.

PHYSICAL EXAMINATION

On inspection the boy was sitting up and in obvious respiratory distress. He demonstrated a frequent brassy cough, and inspiratory stridor was clearly present. He was flushed, anxious, gasping for air, and crying quietly. His blood pressure was 110/70, apical heart rate 160 bpm, respiratory rate 58/min, and temperature normal. Chest examination showed obvious intercostal and supraclavicular retractions. Palpation and percussion were unremarkable. Normal but diminished breath sounds were auscultated. His oxygen saturation measured by pulse oximetry (SpO_2) while he was on an oxygen mask was 88%. The attending physician ordered a chest x-ray.

Response 1

Based on the previous clinical information, write your SOAP in the following space.

S _____

_____

O _____

_____

_____

_____

_____

_____

_____

_____

A _____

_____

_____

_____

_____

_____

_____

_____

_____

_____

Response 1–cont'd

P _____

_____

_____

_____

_____

_____

I HOUR LATER

Despite the treatment administered the patient still appeared to be in respiratory distress. He had intercostal and supraclavicular retractions. His inspiratory stridor showed no change, and his cough was still frequent and brassy sounding. In a hoarse voice he said he wanted to go home. His vital signs were as follows: blood pressure 146/88, apical heart rate 155 bpm, respiratory rate 63/min, and temperature normal. His chest x-ray showed a subglottic haziness (Fig. 25-1, with a close-up of the neck region of Fig. 25-1 pictured in Fig. 25-2). Breath sounds were normal but diminished. His SpO_2 was 90%.

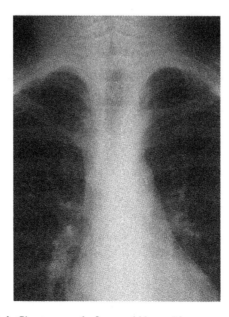

Fig. 25-1 Chest x-ray of a 3-year-old boy with croup syndrome.

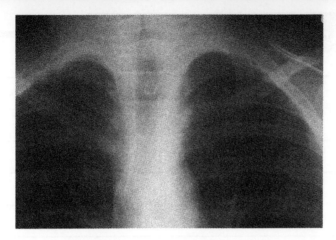

Fig. 25-2 Close-up x-ray of the boy's neck.

Response 2

Based on the previous clinical information, write your SOAP in the following space.

S _____

_____

O _____

_____

_____

_____

_____

_____

_____

_____

A _____

_____

_____

_____

Response 2–cont'd

P _____

CHRISTMAS EVE

At 1:30 AM the physician called the respiratory care consult service to evaluate the patient's respiratory status and make recommendations regarding the patient's discharge status. The respiratory care practitioner found the boy sitting up in his bed coloring. The patient nodded when asked whether he felt better. Inspiratory stridor no longer was audible, and intercostal or supraclavicular retractions no longer could be seen. His blood pressure was 125/80, apical heart rate 89 bpm, and respiratory rate 15/min. Breath sounds were normal. His SpO_2 was 97%.

Response 3

Based on the previous clinical information, write your SOAP in the following space.

S _____

O _____

Continued

Response 3–cont'd

A

P

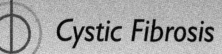

Cystic Fibrosis

26

ADMITTING HISTORY

A 27-year-old man has a long history of respiratory problems due to cystic fibrosis. Even though his medical records are incomplete, he reported on admission that his parents told him that he had suffered several episodes of pneumonia during his early years. He is an adopted child and therefore does not know his biologic family history. His parents are actively involved in his general care, which entails the home-care suggestions or therapeutic procedures presented by the pulmonary rehabilitation team. He takes supplemental multivitamins and timed-release pancreatic enzymes regularly, as prescribed by his doctor.

During his teens he had fewer respiratory symptoms than he has today and was able to live a relatively normal life. During that time he took up water-skiing and became proficient in the slalom event. He is known to most of his associates as a "wonder." Although he qualifies for disability because of his continual shortness of breath, he is able to do various small jobs, which always relate to water-skiing. He is well known throughout the water-skiing circuit as an excellent chief judge at national and regional tournaments. In addition, he is a certified driver for jump-trick and slalom events and recently has become involved in selling water-ski tournament ropes and handles, which provides him with a small additional income.

Over the past 3 years his cough has become more persistent and increasingly productive, with about a cupful of sputum noted daily. Over the same period he has noted intermittent hemoptysis and become short of breath when climbing stairs. Even though the man has a normal appetite, he has lost a great deal of weight over the past 2 years. On admission he denied experiencing any recent changes in bowel habits despite his weight loss but said that he has noticed a tendency to pass rather pale stools. Much to the chagrin of his doctor, 3 years ago he began smoking about 10 cigarettes a day, his reason being that the cigarettes help him cough up the sputum.

PHYSICAL EXAMINATION

On examination the patient appeared pale, cyanotic, and thin. He had a barrel chest and was using his accessory muscles of respiration. Clubbing of the fingers was present. He demonstrated a frequent, productive cough. His sputum was sweet smelling, thick, and yellow-green. His neck veins were distended, and he showed

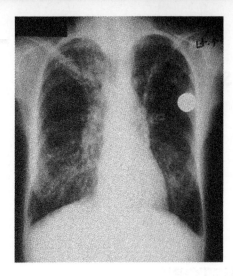

Fig. 26-1   Chest x-ray of a 27-year-old man with cystic fibrosis.

mild-to-moderate peripheral edema. He stated that he had not been this short of breath in a long time.

He had a blood pressure of 142/90, a heart rate of 108 bpm, and a respiratory rate of 28/min, he was afebrile. Palpation of the chest was unremarkable. Expiration was prolonged. Hyperresonant notes were elicited bilaterally during percussion. Auscultation revealed diminished breath sounds and heart sounds. Crackles and rhonchi were heard throughout both lung fields.

His chart showed that during his last medical checkup (about 10 months before this admission) a pulmonary function test (PFT) was conducted. Results revealed moderate-to-severe airway obstruction. No blood gases were analyzed.

His chest x-ray on this admission revealed hyperlucent lung fields, depressed hemidiaphragms, and right ventricular enlargement (Fig. 26-1). His arterial blood gas values (ABGs) on 1.5 L/min oxygen by nasal cannula were as follows: pH 7.51, $Paco_2$ 58 mm Hg, HCO_3^- 43 mmol/L, and Pao_2 66 mm Hg. His hemoglobin oxygen saturation measured by pulse oximetry (Spo_2) was 94%.

Response 1

Based on the previous information, write your SOAP in the following space.

S _____

_____

O _____

_____

Response 1–cont'd

A

P

48 HOURS AFTER ADMISSION

The respiratory therapist from the consult service noted that the patient was again in respiratory distress. The man stated that he could not get enough air to sleep even 10 minutes. He appeared cyanotic and was using his accessory muscles of respiration. His vital signs were as follows: blood pressure 147/95, heart rate 117 bpm, respiratory rate 32/min, and temperature 37° C (98.6° F).

He coughed frequently, and although his cough was weak, he produced large amounts of thick, green sputum. Hyperresonant notes were produced during percussion over both lung fields. On auscultation, breath sounds and heart sounds were diminished. Crackles, rhonchi, and wheezing were heard throughout both lung fields. No recent chest x-ray was available. A sputum culture confirmed the presence of *Pseudomonas aeruginosa*. His SpO_2 was 92% and his ABGs were as follows: pH 7.55, $PaCO_2$ 54 mm Hg, HCO_3^- 45 mmol/L, and PaO_2 57 mm Hg.

Response 2

Based on the previous information, write your SOAP in the following space.

S _____

_____

O _____

_____

_____

_____

_____

_____

_____

_____

A _____

_____

_____

_____

_____

Response 2–cont'd

P

64 HOURS AFTER ADMISSION

The respiratory care practitioner noted that the patient was in obvious respiratory distress. The patient indicated he could not find a position to breathe comfortably. He appeared cyanotic and was pursed-lip breathing, using his accessory muscles of respiration. His vital signs were as follows: blood pressure 145/90, heart rate 120 bpm, respiratory rate 22/min, and oral temperature 38° C (100.5° F). Palpation was normal, but bilateral hyperresonant percussion notes were elicited. Auscultation revealed crackles, rhonchi, and wheezing bilaterally. No recent chest x-ray was available. His SpO_2 was 65%, and his ABGs were as follows: pH 7.33, $PaCO_2$ 79 mm Hg, HCO_3^- 41 mmol/L, and PaO_2 37 mm Hg.

Response 3

Based on the previous information, write your SOAP in the following space.

S

O

Response 3—cont'd

A

P

PART XIII

Other Important Topics

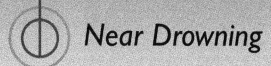

Near Drowning

27

ADMITTING HISTORY

An 18-year-old white man was part of a 300-student graduating class from a Colorado high school in the foothills of the Rocky Mountains. Graduation took place in late May. The day before the graduation ceremony, about 80 students spent most of the day and evening in the mountains, roasting a pig, playing volleyball, and consuming large quantities of beer. Reports later stated that seven empty kegs of beer were tied down in one pickup truck alone.

Driving down the narrow and curving mountain road was difficult to do sober during daylight, let alone at night with an elevated blood alcohol level. Unfortunately the man, who was intoxicated, chose to drive his pickup home. His girlfriend and best friend were passengers in the vehicle. Several other cars and trucks filled with students also were traveling down the mountain at the same time. About 10 miles from town the man's truck suddenly swerved off the road, went down a 7.5 m (25 foot) embankment, and plunged into a river. Within seconds the truck was completely submerged. Reports later established that the water temperature was about 13° C (55° F).

The man's girlfriend and best friend swam to safety. He did not. He was not breathing when he was pulled from the wreckage by three students from a truck following his. The man was thought to have been trapped underneath the water for approximately 10 minutes. Cardiopulmonary resuscitation (CPR) was administered by two students who recently had completed a first-aid course. Another student called 911 on his cellular phone.

When the paramedics arrived, the patient was unconscious, and his pupils were fixed and dilated. No external evidence of head trauma was present. He had a pulse but no respirations. An oral airway was inserted, and the patient was manually ventilated with 100% oxygen attached to an E-tank. En route to the hospital the patient's wet clothing was removed, and he was wrapped in several warm blankets. His vital signs were as follows: blood pressure 126/84, heart rate 118 bpm, respiratory rate 26/min, and rectal temperature 31° C (88.7° F). His oxygen saturation measured by pulse oximetry (SpO$_2$) was 91%.

On arrival in the emergency department the patient was no longer being manually ventilated by the paramedics. He demonstrated a rapid, gasping breathing pattern. He was semiconscious and thrashing around. Despite being on a nonrebreathing mask, he appeared cyanotic. His pupils were equal and sluggishly reactive.

Except for some minor bruises and abrasions on his lower extremities, no traumatic injuries were apparent.

His vital signs were as follows: blood pressure 137/89, heart rate 122 bpm, respiratory rate 28/min, and rectal temperature 32.3° C (90.3° F). Palpation of the chest was unremarkable. Over the lung bases, dull percussion notes were elicited and fine crackles were auscultated. His arterial blood gas values (ABGs) were as follows: pH 7.11, $Paco_2$ 72 mm Hg, HCO_3^- 18 mmol/L, and Pao_2 36 mm Hg. The patient's Spo_2 was 57%. Near drowning was written as the diagnosis in the patient's chart.

The patient was intubated, transferred to the intensive care unit, and placed on a mechanical ventilator. His initial ventilator settings were as follows: assist/control mode, 12 breaths per minute, tidal volume 750 ml, and Fio_2 0.50. A portable chest x-ray showed that the endotracheal tube was positioned correctly, and bilateral patchy infiltrates were noted in both lower lobes (Fig. 27-1). Approximately 12 minutes after the patient was placed on the ventilator, his ABGs were as follows: pH 7.23, $Paco_2$ 51 mm Hg, HCO_3^- 19 mmol/L, and Pao_2 54 mm Hg. His Spo_2 was 84%.

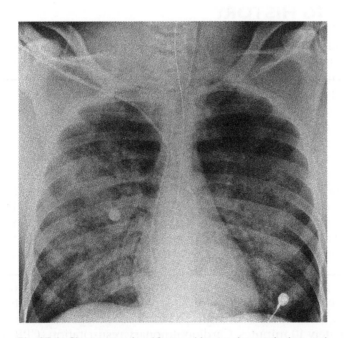

Fig. 27-1 Chest x-ray of an 18-year-old man who nearly drowned.

Response 1

Based on the previous information, write your SOAP in the following space.

S _____

_____

Response 1 – cont'd

O

A

P

45 MINUTES LATER

The patient was sedated and quiet. An arterial catheter and intravenous line were in place. No further changes had been made in the ventilator setting. His vital signs were as follows: blood pressure 125/86, heart rate 130 bpm, and rectal temperature 33.4° C (92.3° F). The patient's chest assessment data had deteriorated since admission; dull percussion notes now were elicited throughout both lung fields, and more prominent crackles and rhonchi were heard over both lungs. A moderate amount of frothy, white sputum, occasionally streaked with yellow mucus and possible food chunks was being suctioned from the patient's endotracheal tube. Because a recent chest x-ray was not available, a stat chest x-ray was ordered by the head nurse. His ABGs were as follows: pH 7.53, $Paco_2$ 28 mm Hg, HCO_3^- 21 mmol/L, and Pao_2 56 mm Hg. His Spo_2 was 89%.

Response 2

Based on the previous information, write your SOAP in the following space.

S _____

_____

O _____

_____

_____

_____

_____

_____

_____

A _____

_____

_____

_____

_____

Response 2–cont'd

P _____

_____

_____

_____

_____

_____

_____

10 HOURS LATER

The patient's cardiopulmonary status remained critical. He was still heavily sedated, and his skin was cool to the touch and appeared cyanotic. His vital signs were as follows: blood pressure 100/60, heart rate 150 bpm, and rectal temperature 39.5° C (103° F). Despite aggressive suctioning and anterior chest percussion and drainage, crackles and rhonchi were now abundant throughout all lung fields. Frothy, pink secretions were difficult to keep from the patient's endotracheal tube.

Large doses of diuretics and cardiac agents had been used for some time now, but with marginal results. The patient's pupils again were fixed and dilated. A neurologist had been called in for consultation. A recent portable chest x-ray revealed fluffy infiltrate throughout both lung fields that was consistent with a pulmonary edema pattern. His ABGs were as follows: pH 7.35, $PaCO_2$ 37 mm Hg, HCO_3^- 23 mmol/L, and PaO_2 47 mm Hg. His SpO_2 was 80%.

Response 3

Based on the previous information, write your SOAP in the following space.

S _____

_____

Continued

Response 3—cont'd

O

A

P

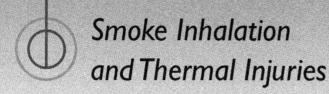

Smoke Inhalation and Thermal Injuries

ADMITTING HISTORY

A 46-year-old white man was rescued by the fire department from his two-story home. A taxicab operator driving by the man's home at about 4 AM saw the house engulfed with fire and smoke. He reported the fire to his dispatcher, who in turn called the fire department. The fire department arrived about 25 minutes later. Neighbors reported that a single man lived in the house. Approximately 5 minutes later a fireman exited the house carrying a middle-aged man. He had been found unconscious in bed in a smoke- and flame-filled room.

The patient displayed agonal respirations. He is known to be a three-pack-per-day cigarette smoker. His left leg, left arm, and anterior trunk were burned severely. No burns were noted on his head or neck. The paramedics immediately inserted an oral airway and started to manually ventilate the patient with 100% oxygen. A pulse was palpable, and the man was quickly transferred to the ambulance. En route to the hospital an intravenous infusion of Ringer's lactate solution was started, an ampule of bicarbonate administered, and the remainder of the patient's pajamas cut away.

The patient was unresponsive to deep pain. His pupils were dilated, but both reacted slowly to intense light. His nasal hairs were singed, and he had a frequent, loose-sounding cough. After each coughing episode the paramedics suctioned a small amount of coal-colored sputum from his oral and nasal pharynx. His vital signs en route to the hospital were as follows: blood pressure 153/98 and heart rate 109 bpm. His oxygen saturation measured by pulse oximetry (SpO_2) was 97%.

On arrival in the emergency room the patient was immediately intubated and placed on mechanical ventilation. Most of his burns were classified as second degree. His left foot had third-degree burns. After the burns were debrided and dressed, the patient was transferred to the intensive care unit. The initial ventilator settings were as follows: assist/control mode, 14 breaths per minute, tidal volume 800 ml, +5 cm H_2O continuous positive airway pressure (CPAP), and FIO_2 1.0.

Approximately 20 minutes after the patient was placed on the mechanical ventilator, his blood pressure was 157/105 and his heart rate 112 bpm. He did not exhibit spontaneous ventilations. His skin appeared cherry-red. Frothy, sooty-appearing sputum was suctioned from the endotracheal tube. Crackles and rhonchi were auscultated over both lung fields. A portable chest x-ray revealed bilateral diffuse pulmonary infiltrates consistent with noncardiogenic pulmonary edema (Fig. 28-1). The patient's arterial blood gas values (ABGs) were as follows: pH 7.52, $PaCO_2$ 28 mm Hg, HCO_3^- 22 mmol/L, and PaO_2 202 mm Hg. His SpO_2 was 98%. His carboxyhemoglobin level (COHb) was 30%. No cyanide was detected in the patient's blood.

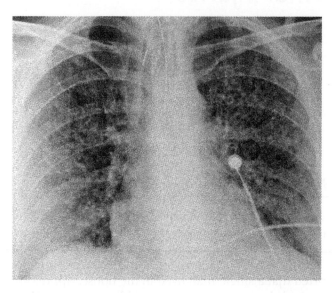

Fig. 28-1 Chest x-ray of a 46-year-old man who suffered smoke inhalation and burns.

Response 1

Based on the previous information, write your SOAP in the following space.

S _____

_____

O _____

_____

_____

_____

_____

_____

Response 1—cont'd

A _____

_____

_____

_____

_____

_____

_____

_____

P _____

_____

_____

_____

_____

_____

24 HOURS AFTER ADMISSION

The patient was still unconscious, and his cardiopulmonary status was unstable. His COHb was 20% after his first hyperbaric oxygen (HBO) treatment. A pulmonary arterial catheter and central venous pressure line had been inserted. His pulmonary capillary wedge pressure (PCWP) was 20 cm H_2O. The patient's blood pressure was 127/88, and his heart rate was 82 bpm. His total respiratory rate (on assist/control ventilation) was 30/min, and he was afebrile. All other hemodynamic indices were normal. His skin still appeared cherry-red, and frothy, sooty secretions were still being suctioned from his endotracheal tube every 15 or 20 minutes.

Crackles and rhonchi were still auscultated over both lung fields. A recent portable chest x-ray showed that the endotracheal tube was in a good position but that the pulmonary infiltrates were becoming worse. The patient's ABGs were as follows: pH 7.29, $Paco_2$ 37 mm Hg, HCO_3^- 18 mmol/L, and Pao_2 63 mm Hg.

Response 2

Based on the previous information, write your SOAP in the following space.

S _____

_____

O _____

_____

_____

_____

_____

_____

_____

A _____

_____

_____

_____

_____

_____

_____

_____

P _____

_____

_____

_____

_____

_____

4 DAYS AFTER ADMISSION

The patient was conscious but sedated, and his burns were starting to heal nicely; no signs of infection were present. His cardiopulmonary status, however, continued to be unstable. Furosemide (Lasix) had been used on and off for diuresis in the interval, but despite this action, he had gained 6 lb since the assessment 3 days earlier. He remained intubated on assist/control ventilation. Large amounts of thick, gray and yellow secretions were being suctioned from his endotracheal tube. A sputum culture was positive for *Pseudomonas*.

A recent chest x-ray showed infiltrates throughout both lung fields, which suggested severe pulmonary edema and atelectasis. In addition, the radiologist also believed that the patient was developing adult respiratory distress syndrome (ARDS). Shortly after the radiologist's report arrived, the respiratory therapist assisted the physician in a therapeutic bronchoscopy. Numerous eschars and mucus plugs were suctioned from the tracheobronchial tree.

The patient's skin no longer appeared red. A few hours earlier his hemodynamic indices had indicated a moderate increase in his pulmonary vascular resistance (PVR) and systemic vascular resistance (SVR) and a moderate decrease in all other parameters. The PWCP was normal. Fluid resuscitation was administered, and all the hemodynamic indices returned to normal. His ABGs were as follows: pH 7.25, $Paco_2$ 39 mm Hg, HCO_3^- 18 mmol/L, and Pao_2 37 mm Hg. After his second HBO treatment his COHb was 10%. The physician prescribed a repeat hyperbaric treatment despite the COHb measurement because the Pao_2 was so low and lactic acidosis was present.

Response 3

Based on the previous information, write your SOAP in the following space.

S _____

_____

O _____

_____

_____

_____

_____

_____

_____

_____

Continued

Response 3—cont'd

A _____

_____

_____

_____

_____

_____

_____

P _____

_____

_____

_____

_____

_____

Postoperative Atelectasis

29

ADMITTING HISTORY

A 43-year-old woman was admitted to the hospital for an exploratory thoracotomy to diagnose and excise a 1.5-cm pulmonary nodule that had resisted diagnosis by bronchoscopy and percutaneous needle biopsy. She has been a registered nurse for the past 15 years and up until about a year ago was the director of nursing at the admitting hospital. For the past 4 months she has been working the night shift as a general floor nurse in a nursing home owned by the hospital. Although she is considered an attractive woman, her general appearance over the last several years has progressively declined. For the past 3 years she has rapidly moved from a normal, healthy weight to obesity.

Over the last 6 months she almost always has worn one of the same three outfits, gone without makeup, and increased her smoking from one to two and a half packs of cigarettes a day. Her general hygiene has been poor, and her hair often appears dirty. Her estranged husband reported that she has been depressed for the past year or so. He described how he unsuccessfully suggested that they both see a marriage counselor. Frustrated, he moved into his brother's apartment a few miles away from his wife. Despite these events, they continue to speak to each other regularly.

The patient was seen in the preoperative education area before her surgery. Her forced vital capacity (FVC) was normal, but her forced expiratory volume in 1 second (FEV_1) was 50% of the predicted value. She frequently generated a spontaneous, strong cough, producing moderate amounts of yellow sputum. She was instructed on the use of aerosolized medication therapy via metered dose inhaler (MDI) and deep breathing and coughing (C&DB) techniques. Her attention span, however, was poor, and she continually sang words of praise and recognition to every employee who passed her room. She also flooded the respiratory therapist with "aren't you wonderful" phrases as the therapist tried to ask her to demonstrate the various techniques she would be required to perform after her surgery.

After her surgery, while in the postanesthesia area, she continually used foul language and threatened to have everyone fired. Her physician ordered a sedative and then transferred her to the postoperative unit. Over the next 2 hours the patient's general respiratory status declined. Concerned, the primary nurse paged the physician. Busy in another part of the hospital, the physician requested a respiratory care consult.

PHYSICAL EXAMINATION (TIME: 1330)

The respiratory care practitioner noted that the patient was awake and in obvious respiratory distress. Her vital signs were as follows: blood pressure 185/90, heart rate 130 bpm, respiratory rate 35/min, and temperature normal. She demonstrated a frequent spontaneous, weak cough. She often expectorated a moderate amount of yellow sputum during a coughing episode. She appeared cyanotic and quickly stated, "Damn, my gut really hurts, . . . and I can't seem to get any air."

Over the left lower lung, diminished breath sounds were noted. Bronchial breath sounds and dull percussion notes were noted over the right lower lung. The nurse indicated that the patient's incentive spirometry (IS) volume was only about 40% of her preoperative value (when she could get the patient to attempt to use the device). Her oxygen saturation measured by pulse oximetry (SpO_2) on a 2 L/min oxygen nasal cannula was 77%. Arterial blood gas values (ABGs) obtained by the respiratory care practitioner were as follows: pH 7.57, $PaCO_2$ 23 mm Hg, HCO_3^- 21 mmol/L, and PaO_2 43 mm Hg. No recent chest x-ray was available. As the therapist documented the data, the patient's physician entered the room and stated, "I'll do anything to keep this patient off the ventilator. Keep me informed." The physician then prescribed some medication for the patient's pain and quickly left the room.

Response 1

Based on the previous information, write your SOAP in the following space.

S _____

_____

O _____

_____

_____

_____

_____

_____

_____

_____

_____

Response 1—cont'd

A _____

_____

_____

_____

_____

_____

_____

_____

P _____

_____

_____

_____

_____

_____

_____

I DAY AFTER SURGERY

Despite the patient's need for aggressive respiratory care, she was generally unco-operative or unwilling to tolerate various treatment modalities. She had not been transferred to the intensive care unit (ICU). Her skin was blue, cool, and damp. Her eyes were closed, and she was unresponsive to questions. She still demonstrated a weak cough every few minutes. Although sputum retention was suspected, none was actually seen; the patient was believed to be swallowing any sputum produced. Her vital signs were as follows: blood pressure 188/100, heart rate 135 bpm, respiratory rate 36/min, and rectal temperature 38.1° C (100.6° F).

On chest assessment dull percussion notes, bronchial breath sounds, and crackles were noted over the right middle and both lower lobes. A portable chest x-ray revealed that she had mild atelectasis in the right middle and both lower lobes. Air bronchograms also were noted in this area (Fig. 29-1). Her SpO_2 was 72%. Her ABGs were as follows: pH 7.55, Pa_{CO_2} 29 mm Hg, HCO_3^- 22 mmol/L, and Pa_{O_2} 46 mm Hg.

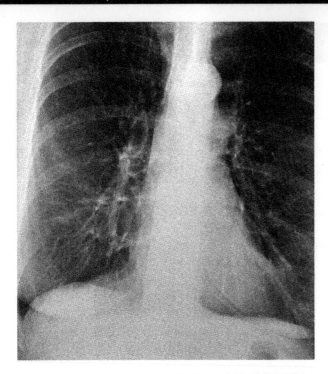

Fig. 29-1 Chest x-ray of a 43-year-old woman who developed postoperative atelectasis.

Response 2

Based on the previous information, write your SOAP in the following space.

S _____

_____

O _____

_____

_____

_____

_____

_____

_____

_____

_____

_____

Response 2 – cont'd

A _____

_____

_____

_____

_____

_____

_____

_____

P _____

_____

_____

_____

_____

_____

_____

7 HOURS LATER

A therapeutic bronchoscopy was performed in the ICU. The patient was not intubated.

The respiratory care practitioner on the pulmonary consult team found the patient in obvious respiratory distress. Her skin was cyanotic, cool, and damp. She stated, "I think I'm dying." No cough was observed at this time. No right-sided chest excursion could be seen, and her trachea was deviated to the right.

Her vital signs were as follows: blood pressure 192/90, heart rate 142 bpm, respiratory rate 20/min, and oral temperature 37.3° C (99.1° F). Bronchial breath sounds, crackles, and dull percussion notes were found over the right middle and lower lobes. Dull percussion notes and no breath sounds were noted over the left lower lobe. Her SpO_2 was 62%. Her ABGs were as follows: pH 7.26, $PaCO_2$ 53 mm Hg, HCO_3^- 22 mmol/L, and PaO_2 37 mm Hg.

Response 3

Based on the previous information, write your SOAP in the following space.

S _____

_____

O _____

_____

_____

_____

_____

_____

_____

_____

A _____

_____

_____

_____

_____

_____

_____

_____

P _____

_____

_____

_____

_____

_____

_____

KEY POINT QUESTIONS

For Postoperative Atelectasis (DRG* 101/102)

1. Basic Concept Formation
   a. What should happen to the volume of an alveolus, lobule, or lobe of the lung if it becomes *airless?*
   b. What would be the effect on oxygenation of pulmonary capillary blood passing such an area?
   c. Name *two simple causes* for atelectasis.
   d. Would coughing, deep breathing, and secretion removal *reverse* some of this pathologic process?
2. Database Formation
   a. What is your *vision of the pathologic process* of pulmonary atelectasis?
   b. Which *pathophysiologic mechanisms* are activated as a result of these anatomic alterations?
   c. Are any portions of the *airway model* (Fig. 1-14) abnormal in usual cases of atelectasis?
   d. What changes might be expected if atelectasis is left untreated or allowed to *worsen?*
   e. What are the most common *causes* of atelectasis?
   f. What are the *goals of therapy* for such patients?
   g. Which *standard therapist-driven protocols (TDPs)* should achieve these purposes?
      1. List the potential *adverse effects* of each protocol you have selected.
      2. How would you *monitor* the beneficial or adverse effects of the therapies you have selected?
3. Assessment
   a. Did this patient's history suggest that she might develop atelectasis?
   b. Did this patient initially or subsequently demonstrate any evidence of the *clinical manifestations* of atelectasis? If so, what were they?
   c. Did this patient initially demonstrate any evidence of the *pathophysiologic alterations* commonly associated with atelectasis?
   d. Which specific clinical manifestations did this patient demonstrate that helped you decide on the *severity* of her condition?
4. Application
   a. *Sputum induction* (was/was not) indicated because _____ .
   b. *Oxygen therapy* (was/was not) indicated because _____ .
   c. *Bronchial hygiene therapy* (was/was not) indicated because _____ .
   d. *Hyperinflation therapy* (was/was not) indicated because _____ .
   e. *Aerosolized medication therapy* (was/was not) indicated because _____
      _____ .
   f. *Mechanical ventilation* (was/was not) indicated in this case because
      _____ .
   g. *Pulmonary rehabilitation* (was/was not) indicated because _____ .
5. Evaluation
   a. What are the expected results of each therapy you have selected? Are complications expected from these modalities?
   b. How should you monitor the patient's response to each modality?

---

*DRG, *Diagnosis-related group.*   *Continued*

KEY POINT QUESTIONS—cont'd

    c. How can you up-regulate the intensity and/or frequency of each modality as needed?

    d. What are the advantages and disadvantages of each treatment modality that you have selected?

    e. What do you do if the patient improves?

    f. What do you do if she doesn't?

6. Boundary Awareness

    a. How would you know if *this* patient's condition does not improve or worsens?

    b. When should you ask a supervisor for help?

    c. When should you call the patient's physician?

Suggested SOAP Responses, Case Discussions, and Key Point Answers

The SOAP responses* presented throughout Appendix I are intended only as a guide. Depending on the specific case and severity of the clinical manifestations, other assessments and treatment selections may be appropriate. In addition, the clinical manifestations in the parentheses to the right of each assessment likely would not appear in the patient's chart. They are presented in this discussion only to justify each assessment.

Chapter 2   Chronic Bronchitis

Response 1

S: "I'm unable to breathe. I can't inhale deep enough to cough up secretions, and my stomach is upset."

O: Vitals: BP 190/115, HR 125, RR 30, T 37° C (98.6° F); barrel chest, labored breathing, use of accessory muscles, digital clubbing, cyanosis, and pitting ankle edema (1+); copious thick, yellow sputum; chest hyperresonant, with rhonchi heard bilaterally; CXR: lungs clear, air trapping, and depressed diaphragm; Hct 58%. COHb 6%; ABGs (room air): pH 7.53, $PaCO_2$ 56, HCO_3^- 33, PaO_2 43

A: • Acute exacerbation of chronic bronchitis (general presentation, sputum, vital signs, ABGs)
   • Increased work of breathing (increased heart rate, blood pressure, and respiratory rate)
   • Excessive airway secretions (sputum, rhonchi)
       Infection likely (thick, yellow secretions)
   • Poor ability to mobilize secretions (weak cough)
   • Acute alveolar hyperventilation on top of chronic ventilatory failure (ABGs and history)
       Possible impending ventilatory failure

P: Perform Oxygen Therapy Protocol [e.g., HAFOE (Venturi) mask, FIO_2 0.28]. Begin Aerosolized Medication Therapy Protocol with albuterol MDI, 2 puffs q4h. Start Bronchial Hygiene Therapy Protocol (CPT with PD, C&DB q6h). Obtain sputum sample for culture. Notify physician of impending ventilatory failure. Place intubation equipment and mechanical ventilator on standby. Monitor and evaluate q3h (vital signs: SpO_2, ABG).

---

*C&DB, *Cough and deep breath;* PD, *postural drainage;* CPT, *chest physical therapy;* MDI, *metered dose inhaler;* CPAP, *continuous positive airway pressure;* PEEP, *positive end-expiratory, pressure;* IPPB, *intermittent positive pressure breathing;* IPAB, *intermittent positive airway breathing;* COHb, *carboxyhemoglobin;* BP, *blood pressure;* HR, *heart rate;* RR, *respiratory rate;* T, *temperature;* CXR, *chest x-ray;* PEFR, *peak expiratory flow rate;* PFT, *pulmonary function test;* ABG, *arterial blood gas;* BAL, *bronchoalveolar lavage;* prn, *as required;* q2h, *every 2 hours;* IS, *incentive spirometry;* RML, *right middle lobe;* RLL, *right lower lobe;* RUL, *right upper lobe;* LLL, *left lower lobe;* AFB, *acid-fast bacilli;* D/C, *discontinue;* I&O, *in and out;* SIMV, *synchronized intermittent mechanical ventilation;* FEV_1, *forced expiratory volume in 1 second;* BUN, *blood urea nitrogen;* USN, *ultrasonic nebulization;* CVP, *central venous pressure;* RAP, *right arterial pressure;* $\overline{PA}$, *pulmonary artery pressure;* RVSW1, *right ventricular stroke work index;* PVR, *pulmonary vascular resistance;* PCWP, *pulmonary capillary wedge pressure;* CO, *cardiac output;* SVI, *stroke volume index;* HBO, *hyperbaric oxygen;* FVC, *forced vital capacity;* PIP, *peak inspiratory pressure;* V_T, *total volume;* WBC, *white blood cell.*

Response 2

S: "I'm having a bad period."

O: Vitals: BP 185/135, HR 130, RR 28, T 37° C (98.6° F); use of accessory muscles and pursed-lip breathing; cough weak and productive of large amounts of thick, yellow sputum; bilateral rhonchi; ABGs: pH 7.55, $PaCO_2$ 53, HCO_3^- 32, PaO_2 41; SpO_2: 83%

A: • Continued acute exacerbation of chronic bronchitis without improvement over the past 9 hours (general appearance and clinical data)
   • Continued increased work of breathing (general appearance, elevated heart rate, blood pressure, and respiratory rate)
   • Persistent, excessive airway secretions (sputum, rhonchi)
      Infection likely (yellow sputum)
   • Poor ability to mobilize secretions (weak cough)
   • Acute alveolar hyperventilation on top of chronic ventilatory failure (ABGs and history)
      Impending ventilatory failure

P: Up-regulate Oxygen Therapy Protocol (e.g., FIO_2 0.50). Check ABGs in 15 minutes. Increase Bronchial Hygiene Therapy Protocol (e.g., increasing frequency of CPT and PD to q4h while awake, and once on night shift). Change Aerosolized Medication Protocol (e.g., administer acetylcysteine [Mucomyst] 1.5 cc of 10% solution in 0.5 cc of albuterol in med. neb. q2h; then reevaluate). Notify physician of status. Continue to monitor and evaluate q2h. Check I&O and chart.

Response 3

S: "I'm feeling worse again."

O: Vital signs: BP 150/95, HR 140, RR 25 and shallow, T 37° C (98.6° F); use of accessory muscles of respiration and pursed-lip breathing; cough weak and no sputum production; expiration prolonged; bilateral rhonchi; ABGs: pH 7.28, $PaCO_2$ 105, HCO_3^- 41, PaO_2 44; COHb 2.5%.

A: • Continued exacerbation of chronic bronchitis; unimproved since last evaluation 12 hours earlier (general appearance and clinical data)
   • Excessive airway secretions (rhonchi)
   • Poor ability to mobilize secretions (weak cough)
   • Acute ventilatory failure on top of chronic ventilatory failure (ABGs and history)

P: Page physician stat about ventilatory failure. Retain respiratory therapist on standby for intubation and mechanical ventilation. Begin Mechanical Ventilation Protocol (e.g., initial ventilator settings: FIO_2 0.60, SIMV 12/min, VT 12 ml/kg, PEEP 0). Continue Aerosolized Medication Therapy and Bronchial Hygiene Therapy Protocols as tolerated (e.g., CPT with PD q4h while awake). Monitor and evaluate per ICU standing orders.

DISCUSSION

The return to hospital of a patient with chronic bronchitis who has not complied with therapy is all too familiar to the respiratory care practitioner and physicians. This patient has persisted in smoking cigarettes, refused pulmonary rehabilitation, and now has allowed his personal hygiene to deteriorate.

Shrugging off all this information and discharging him from the emergency room would be easy if a careful assessment were not done. This case presents several worrisome signs of impending respiratory failure, including systemic hypertension, tachycardia, increased work of breathing, decrease in cough efficiency, peripheral edema (suggesting possible cor pulmonale), and signs of pulmonary infection (with yellow sputum), all signs and symptoms (clinical manifestations) of **excessive bronchial secretions** and their associated pathophysiologic mechanisms (i.e., intrapulmonary shunting, hypoxemia, and stimulation of oxygen receptors and the pulmonary reflex response to irritants; see Fig. 1-12). If these warning signs were not enough, his admission blood gases with profound hypoxemia, despite relative alveolar hyperventilation, should stimulate concern. The polycythemia almost certainly reflects chronic hypoxia, and his elevated carboxyhemoglobin level reflects his cigarette smoking.

The **initial assessment** indicates the need for a specific diagnosis of the cause of his pulmonary infection (sputum culture), conservative treatment of his hypoxemia (low-flow oxygen or Venturi mask), and careful monitoring if intubation and mechanical ventilation are indicated. Before the landmark awareness of oxygen-induced hypoventilation, these patients often ended up on ventilators immediately after admission to the hospital. Today the use of low-flow oxygen therapy and noninvasive mechanical ventilation while bronchial hygiene, aerosolized medication, and antibiotic therapy are at work often makes intubation unnecessary, thus permitting a much less expensive and more comfortable recovery. Watchful awareness of both blood pressure and ventilatory status are suggested and certainly indicated.

The **second assessment** occurs in the setting of worsening pulmonary function despite good respiratory care. Clearly the patient slipped from borderline to overt ventilatory failure in the course of his hospitalization. Several points regarding this case are instructive. First, the patient's complaints became increasingly nonspecific as his blood gas values worsened. Indeed in the final assessment the patient's complaints of "feeling worse again" are so nonspecific as to be unhelpful. These nonspecific complaints, combined with his increasing lethargy, suggest acute respiratory failure.

The blood gas values in the **third assessment** confirm acute ventilatory failure on chronic ventilatory failure. At that time the patient's pH was 7.28, and his Pa_{CO_2} was 105 mm Hg. The reader should sense that the patient's cough and subjective complaint of dyspnea in the first assessment is helpful in the making of a diagnosis and should learn that the nonspecific complaints of "I'm having a bad period" and "I'm feeling worse again" really do not help hospital personnel in reaching an accurate assessment as to the nature of the patient's problem.

Another point to note in this case is the installation by the treating therapist of a series of "watchers" that allow for close monitoring of the patient. At first these consist of the therapist's own and the nursing staff's observation, the use of a pulse oximeter, and frequent blood gas analyses. When the patient deteriorates in the last case scenario, he is transferred to the intensive care unit (ICU), where again more minute-to-minute observation is possible. At this juncture therapists would do well to ask themselves the following question: What have I done to ensure that this patient is observed carefully in the course of my interface with him?

Two points in the admitting history are worthy of note. One is, as it turns out, a red herring; the other is not. The red herring is the patient's complaint of mild nausea without abdominal pain or vomiting. The therapist notes that the abdominal examination is negative and goes on to other things. Nausea or anorexia complicating chronic obstructive pulmonary disease (COPD) is so common as to be seen in approximately one third of admitted patients. The cause of the nausea can be peptic ulcer disease, aminophylline toxicity, medication effect, or hypoxic bowel syndrome. This patient was not receiving aminophylline-like drugs as an outpatient and was not taking oral steroids. If he were vomiting or had gastric distension, passing of a nasogastric tube would have been helpful.

That the patient had a recent history of depression, regular cigarette smoking, and disinterest in pulmonary rehabilitation is missed by the treating therapist here. The therapist fails to ascertain whether the patient has a living will or durable medical power of attorney, information he may wish he had pursued if the patient comes to intubation and commitment to ventilator support.

Note that throughout this case the therapist appropriately adjusts the patient's oxygen therapy, bronchial hygiene regimen, and aerosolized medication therapy and presumably uses mucolytics.

This book's purpose is not to specify precisely which treatments need to be ordered. One would imagine, however, that bronchodilator medicines, bronchial hygiene, and mucolytic therapy every 2 hours by an up-draft medication nebulizer might have been used at the start and that these treatments might have been increased to every hour directly before the patient's transfer to the ICU. Similarly and appropriately the therapist's initial suggestion of an oxygen Venturi mask to prevent the patient's CO_2 retention from worsening would have been appropriate. Frequent blood gas analyses are requested. The therapist notes that no acute infiltrates are noted on the chest x-ray film and suspects that the patient's hypoxemia may be chronic, given his elevated hematocrit. The therapist correctly obtains a sputum sample for culture and contacts the attending physician regarding the need for possible intubation.

Discussion with the physician in this case revealed that prior experience with this patient suggested that vigorous respiratory care was enough to keep him from having to go on the ventilator. The therapist and physician agreed that they would observe the patient for a few more hours before making that decision. As it turned out, the patient continued to deteriorate and slipped into frank respiratory failure, ultimately requiring intubation.

The consulting therapist's role here is critical in that the monitors that the therapist sets must be acute enough and repeated frequently enough to allow for evaluation of the patient *essentially every minute.*

In the final scenario, repeating the chest x-ray examination after intubation (to check placement of the endotracheal tube, determine that a pneumothorax or acute pulmonary infiltrate has not developed, and establish a baseline film with the lungs well expanded from deep, respirator-delivered breaths) is a standard practice.

KEY POINT ANSWERS

For Chronic Bronchitis (DRG* 88)

1. Basic Concept Formation
   a. *Cigarette smoking* and, to a much lesser extent, upper airway infections, such as chronic sinusitis, viral infections, and dust and fume exposure
   b. *Yes.* They are the basis for the approved *definition* of the disease: cough productive of sputum for at least 3 months in 2 consecutive years. These symptoms reflect *stimulation of irritant receptors* in the lung by mucus produced by hypersecreting goblet cells and submucous glands.
   c. Normally by a functioning *mucociliary escalator;* rarely by *cough*
   d. *Yes.*
   e. *Absolutely yes,* although the patient may take several months to appreciate the total beneficial effect. (NOTE: The importance of the respiratory care practitioner's role in smoking cessation and other lung health programs cannot be overemphasized.)
2. Database Formation
   a. *Mucus hypersecretion, bronchial obstruction,* and some distal air trapping†
   b. *Airway obstruction, producing relative or absolute shunt physiology,* is activated (see Fig. 1-12). In addition, stimulation of oxygen receptors, the irritant (cough) reflex, and alveolar hyperinflation account for some of the clinical manifestations.
   c. The *lumen* (secretions) and *wall* (infection and inflammation) (see Fig. 1-14)
   d. *Cyanosis, digital clubbing, erythrocytosis, and cor pulmonale with peripheral edema*
   e. *Goals:* Reduce inflammation, reduce viscosity of sputum, effect expectoration of mucus, and treat hypoxemia and CO_2 retention. Relieve bronchospasm if present.
   f. *Treatment (TDP selection),* as follows:
      1. *Bronchial Hygiene Therapy Protocol* (see Protocol 1-2 and Fig. 1-12): For lumen obstruction (see Fig. 1-14), perform deep breathing and coughing, suction, airway (aerosol) and systemic hydration, and bronchoscopy.
      2. *Aerosolized Medication Protocol* (see Protocol 1-4 and Fig. 1-11): When wall abnormalities are present (see Fig. 1-14), administer systemic antibiotics (physician ordered), antiinflammatory agents, or decongestants (rarely).
      3. *Pulmonary Rehabilitation Protocol* (see Fig. 1-13): For supporting structures, perform pursed-lip breathing exercises.
      4. Perform *Oxygen Therapy Protocol* (see Protocol 1-1) as needed for hypoxemia.

Protocol	Expected Outcomes	Possible Adverse Effects	Monitors
Bronchial Hygiene (see Protocol 1-2)	Increased sputum clearance, decreased wheezing	Rare; percussion and PD possibly not be tolerated	Auscultation, sputum findings
Oxygen Therapy (see Protocol 1-1)	Improved hypoxemia	CO_2 retention	SpO_2, ABGs

3. Assessment
   a. *Yes;* dyspnea, productive cough, obstructive physiology on pulmonary function tests (PFTs), physical signs of air trapping, rhonchi, clubbing, hypoxemia, CO_2 retention, and polycythemia.

DRG, Diagnosis-related group.
†*See color plate 2 in Des Jardins T, Burton GG. Clinical manifestations & assessment of respiratory disease, ed 4, St Louis, 2002, Mosby.*

Continued

    b. *Yes.* His ABGs suggest shunt physiology. His polycythemia and edema reflect chronic hypoxemia. His PFT data suggest airway obstruction and air trapping. This information was confirmed by his chest physical examination.

    c. The *most worrisome manifestations on admission were* pitting leg edema, tachycardia, hypertension, significant hypoxemia, and moderate CO_2 retention.

4. Application

    a. *Oxygen therapy was* indicated because of the profound hypoxemia and signs of cor pulmonale.

    b. *Monitoring* of heart rate and rhythm, electrocardiogram (ECG) morphology, and pulse oximetry *were* indicated because of the hypoxia. Frequent *level of consciousness checks and sputum volume and consistency* checks also were indicated.

    c. Aerosolized medication therapy *was* indicated because of the patient's increased work of breathing.

    d. *Bronchial hygiene therapy was* indicated because of the patient's diagnosis (chronic bronchitis), specifically because of his thick, tenacious secretions.

    e. *Percussion and PD were* indicated (see 4.d).

    f. If smoking cessation instruction and assistance are part of it, *pulmonary rehabilitation should* be involved in this patient's care. His use of oxygen and metered does inhaler (MDI) aerosol therapy should be initiated and evaluated by the pulmonary rehabilitation team.

5. Evaluation

    a. See answer 2.g.

    b. See answer 2.g.

    c. *Limits* of suggested therapies, as follows:

      1. *Aerosolized medication therapy:* At the extreme end, bronchodilators may be administered continuously in cases of severe bronchospasm (see Chapter 5).

      2. *Bronchial hygiene therapy:* Mucolytic therapy can be given via aerosol every 2 to 3 hours. Suctioning can be done every 2 to 3 minutes. Percussion and PD are usually not tolerated for more than 30 minutes every 4 hours. Therapeutic bronchoscopy may be done each shift if necessary.

      3. *Oxygen therapy:* Upper limit of mask therapy FIO_2 (to $FIO_2 = 1.0$) is determined by ABG analysis and worsening of the patient's CO_2 retention.

    d. *Advantages and disadvantages of treatment modalities:* All are relatively inexpensive (except bronchoscopy) and, with the cautions outlined in answer 2.g, relatively safe. The most cost-effective approach discussed is *smoking cessation* on the part of the patient.

    e. If the patient *improves,* first reduce the FIO_2, and then reduce the intensity and frequency of aerosolized medication and bronchial hygiene therapy, for example, from every 2 to 3 hours to every 4 to 6 hours to every shift.

    f. If *little initial improvement* is seen, consider intubation and therapeutic bronchoscopy.

6. Boundary Awareness

    a. At the time of the *second* assessment the following parameters had worsened or not improved: *heart rate, blood pressure, and ABGs*

    b. Probably after the *second assessment;* certainly at the time of the *third assessment* because of severe respiratory acidemia

    c. At the time of the *third assessment* in most clinical settings

    d. Unrelieved *dyspnea, tachypnea, tachycardia, worsening ABGs,* failure to produce sputum despite intensive therapy (at the time of the *third assessment*)

    e. See answer 2.g.

Chapter 3   Emphysema

Response 1

S: "I'm so short of breath!"

O: Obvious respiratory distress; vital signs: BP 155/110, HR 95, RR 25, and T 38.3° C (101° F); malnourished (66 kg [146 lb], 180 cm [6 ft] tall); use of accessory muscles of inspiration, pursed-lip breathing; increased anteroposterior chest diameter. Depressed hemidiaphragms and generally diminished breath sounds; expiration prolonged; crackles in right lower lobe; CXR: apical scarring, large bulla in right middle lobe, pulmonary hyperexpansion, right lower lobe infiltrate consistent with pneumonia; cough: weak and productive of small amount of yellow sputum; ABGs (on 1.5 L/min O_2 by nasal cannula): pH 7.59, $Paco_2$ 40, HCO_3^- 37, Pao_2 38

A: • Bronchitic exacerbation of COPD (history, general appearance, ABGs, CXR)
 • Increased work of breathing (increased respiratory rate, blood pressure, and heart rate)
 • Alveolar infiltrate in right lower lobe; presumed lobar pneumonia (CXR, fever)
 • Excessive bronchial secretions and poor ability to mobilize them (yellow sputum and weak cough)
 • Acute alveolar hyperventilation superimposed on chronic ventilatory failure with severe hypoxemia (ABGs and history)
   Impending ventilatory failure
 • Presumed malnutrition

P: Initiate Oxygen Therapy Protocol (e.g., O_2 per nasal cannula at 2.5 lpm) and Bronchial Hygiene Therapy Protocol (e.g., C&DB q2h with supervision; CPT with PD to right lower lobe qid; sputum culture). Begin trial of Aerosolized Medication Protocol (e.g., med. neb. treatments with albuterol 0.5 cc in 2.0 cc NS q2h × 6, then q4h). Have mechanical ventilation on standby. Monitor closely (every hour, vital signs, pulse oximetry, ABGs).

Response 2

S: "My chest feels tighter, and I'm more short of breath."

O: Vital signs: BP 160/115, HR 97, RR 15 and shallow. T 37.8° C (100° F); possibly getting fatigued (e.g., no use of accessory muscles of inspiration); diminished breath sounds; no air entry a possible reason for no crackles in right lower lobe; ABGs: pH 7.28, $Paco_2$ 82, HCO_3^- 36, Pao_2 41; Spo_2 68%

A: • Continued increase in respiratory distress and fatigue (blood pressure, heart rate, shallow respiratory rate, no use of accessory muscles)
 • Right lower lobe infiltrate (dull percussion notes and admission CXR)
 • Excessive bronchial secretions (thick, yellow, sputum)
 • Acute ventilatory failure superimposed on chronic ventilatory failure with severe hypoxemia ($Paco_2$ higher and pH lower than patient's normal baseline; general patient fatigue)

Continued

Response 2–cont'd

P: Page physician stat. Recommend transfer to ICU. Recommend support via Mechanical Ventilation Protocol (e.g., FIO_2 1.00, VT 900 cc, SIMV 12, PEEP 0). After intubation, perform deep tracheal suction for Gram stain and culture of secretions. Check ABGs 30 minutes after intubation. Continue Aerosolized Medication Protocol as earlier. Add mucolytic (e.g., acetylcysteine 2 cc of 20% solution q6h). Continue Bronchial Hygiene Therapy Protocol as earlier. Monitor closely and evaluate per ICU standing orders. Plan to review nutrition consult.

DISCUSSION

Emphysema is a slowly progressive *destructive* process involving lung parenchyma. In the case of panacinar (panlobular) emphysema the loss of pulmonary function may be as much as 60 to 100 cc of forced expiratory volume in 1 second (FEV_1) per year. More rapid declines in pulmonary function are accompanied by conditions known to exacerbate chronic obstructive pulmonary disease (COPD; e.g., acute bronchitis, pneumonia, pneumothorax). In this case the patient's fever, history of a flulike syndrome, crackles in the right lower lobe, and a right lower lobe infiltrate on the chest x-ray all point to acute pneumonia as reason for his deterioration. A correct response in this case was the rapid obtaining of a Gram stain and culture of the sputum. In addition, the patient was coughing up large amounts of thick, yellow sputum in the second assessment. Thus not only did the patient demonstrate many clinical manifestations associated with **distal airway and alveolar weakening** (see Fig. 1-13), but also the patient's condition was compromised by **pulmonic consolidation** (see Fig. 1-9) and **excessive bronchial secretions** (see Fig. 1-12).

A "red herring" in this case is the patient's earlier reported failure to improve with aerosolized medication therapy. Any exacerbation of COPD deserves an in-hospital trial of aggressive bronchial hygiene and aerosolized medication therapy because reversible bronchospasm may be one of the only components of the deterioration that does respond. Accordingly, putting the patient on an up-draft nebulizer treatment with bronchodilator, encouraging deep breathing and coughing, and using mucolytics and systemic hydration are all indicated in this case, even though they were of little use in the past.

A good call for the treating team is to recognize the patient's malnutrition, quantitatively assess it, and bring early professional attention to the condition while he is in the hospital for this pneumonic exacerbation.

That the patient suddenly (at the time of the **second assessment**) slips into acute respiratory failure with significant CO_2 retention is not surprising. In some series of such patients this event occurs more than 50% of the time, despite otherwise judicious use of oxygen and entirely appropriate respiratory care.

The patient previously requested that "no heroics" be used on him, but the attending physician was able to convince the patient to accept a period of mechanical ventilation when his clinical condition deteriorated despite the initial aggressive therapy prescribed. The organism responsible for this exacerbation (pneumococcus) was subsequently identified, and the patient gradually improved as antibiotic therapy and ventilator support were continued for a 10-day hospital stay. The patient was discharged on dietary supplementation and a program of multiple small feedings.

Attention must be drawn to the decreased adventitious breath sounds in the right lower lobe at the *second assessment*. The reader who correctly assumed that these sounds were due to decreased air entry in an airless, possibly obstructed right lower lobe should be congratulated. The fact that the crackles go away within 6 hours of admission does *not* suggest that the patient is improving. Indeed it suggests just the opposite, as evidenced by the patient's deteriorating arterial blood gas values!

Chapter 4   *Bronchiectasis*

Response 1

S: Complaints of constant dyspnea and productive cough

O: Cyanotic, mild digital clubbing; pursed-lip breathing and use of accessory muscles of inspiration; frequent, strong cough; large amounts of foul smelling, yellow-green sputum; vital signs: BP 185/90, HR 110, RR 30, T 37.9° C (100.2° F); bilateral rhonchi and crackles; PFT: mild-to-moderate airway obstruction; bedside PEFR: 325 lpm; ABGs (on 3 L/min O_2 by nasal cannula): pH 7.52, $PaCO_2$ 35, HCO_3^- 27, PaO_2 53; CXR: cystic bronchiectasis, moderate alveolar hyperinflation, increased markings

A: • Respiratory distress and increased work of breathing (general appearance, vital signs, pursed-lip breathing, use of accessory muscles)
   • Excessive bronchial secretions (cough, sputum, rhonchi, and crackles)
      Infection likely (yellow-green sputum)
   • Acute alveolar hyperventilation superimposed on chronic ventilatory failure with mild hypoxemia (ABGs)
   • Possible impending ventilatory failure

P: Initiate Aerosolized Medication Therapy and Bronchial Hygiene Therapy Protocols (e.g., 2 cc 20% acetylcysteine with 0.5 cc albuterol via hand-held nebulizer q6h, followed by C&DB, CPT, and PD to lower lobes. Obtain sputum culture. Perform Oxygen Therapy Protocol: HAFOE at FIO_2 0.40. Check ABGs 1 hour later. Monitor impending ventilatory failure closely (e.g., vital signs, SpO_2 q2h). Train patient in use of flutter valve. Check influenza and pneumonia immunization status.

Response 2

S: "I've been short of breath for several hours."

O: Cyanotic, pursed-lip breathing and use of accessory muscles of respiration; frequent cough, producing large amounts of foul-smelling, bloody, yellow-green secretions; sputum culture: *S. pneumoniae* and *P. aeruginosa*; vital signs: BP 188/95, HR 118, RR 34, T 37° C (98.6° F); flat percussion note over RLL; bilateral rhonchi and crackles; bronchial breath sounds over the RLL; SpO_2 93%; ABGs: pH 7.54, $PaCO_2$ 30, HCO_3^- 28, PaO_2 57; CXR: RLL atelectasis or pneumonic infiltrate

A: • Continued respiratory distress (general appearance, vital signs, pursed-lip breathing, use of accessory muscles)
   • Excessive bronchial secretions (cough, sputum, rhonchi, and crackles)
   • Right lower lobe atelectasis versus pneumonia/consolidation (CXR, bronchial breath sounds)
   • Acute alveolar hyperventilation superimposed on chronic ventilatory failure with mild hypoxemia (ABGs)
   • Possible impending ventilatory failure

Response 2–cont'd

P: Up-regulate Oxygen Therapy Protocol (e.g., increasing F_{IO_2} to 0.5). Check ABGs in 1 hour. Increase Aerosolized Medication and Bronchial Hygiene Protocols (e.g., as previously but q4h around the clock). Start Hyperinflation Therapy Protocol (e.g., incentive spirometry supervised 2×/shift during flutter valve work). Continue close monitoring as before.

Response 3

S: "I'm breathing much better."

O: Strong cough; sputum: moderate amount of thin, clear secretions; vital signs: BP 135/80, HR 85, RR 14, T normal; mild-to-moderate rhonchi and crackles over both lung bases; SpO_2 94%. ABGs: pH 7.48, $PaCO_2$ 49, HCO_3^- 38, PaO_2 66; CXR: opacity no longer present in RLL, no other acute infiltrates

A: • Respiratory distress no longer present (patient's comment, vital signs, ABGs)
  • Bronchial secretions (thin, clear secretions)
      Infection apparently improving
  • Atelectasis/pneumonia improving (CXR, ABGs)
  • Acute alveolar hyperventilation on top of chronic ventilatory failure with mild hypoxemia improving (ABGs)
      Impending ventilatory failure no longer present

P: Down-regulate Oxygen Therapy Protocol (O_2 per nasal cannula @ 2 lpm). Down-regulate Aerosolized Medication and Bronchial Hygiene Therapy Protocols (e.g., reducing med. nebs., C&DB, and PD to 1×/shift, q8h; continue flutter valve). Down-regulate Hyperinflation Therapy Protocol (e.g., IS tid). Reevaluate in AM. If stable, D/C SpO_2 monitoring.

DISCUSSION

Although increasingly rare in clinical practice, bronchiectasis is one of the chronic lung diseases with which the respiratory care practitioner must be familiar. It presents as recurrent pulmonary infections, with variable pulmonary scarring over the years. The pathophysiology is similar to that of cystic fibrosis in that frequently secretions are retained and right-to-left intrapulmonary shunting is present. All the clinical manifestations presented in this case can be trailed easily back to the "clinical scenarios" activated by **excessive bronchial secretions** (Fig. 1-12). In the **second assessment,** flatness to percussion over the right lung base and the auscultation of crackles reflects pneumonic consolidation (Fig. 1-9). **Pneumonic consolidation** and/or **atelectasis** (Fig. 1-8) often *complicate* bronchiectasis.

This patient was already known to the medical center as having bronchiectasis, which resulted in more straightforward care. The bilateral rhonchi and crackles heard on the **first assessment** clearly suggest a need for the aerosolized medication and bronchial hygiene therapy that was performed. This therapy must include postural drainage and percussion therapy, as well as mucolysis. As in all obstructive pulmonary diseases, a trial of bronchodilator therapy in-hospital certainly is not out of order. The sputum often produces organisms such as those seen in this case (*Streptococcus* and *Pseudomonas*), and a sputum culture is appropriate.

Of most concern was the patient's initial blood gas values, which had deteriorated from those 2 years earlier. Most significantly, her drop in PaO_2 from 68 mm Hg on 2 L/min oxygen to 53 mm Hg on 3 L/min was worrisome. Note that no frank pneumonic infiltrate was noted on the initial chest x-ray but that one did appear in the right lower lobe on the third day after admission. This infiltrate could have been from atelectasis due to proximal airway mucus plugging or, alternatively, from an acute pneumonia. The treatments for these conditions are not all that different in that the airway obstruction must be relieved.

Note that on the **second assessment** the patient is developing severe hypoxemia despite any oxygen therapy the therapist would have selected. A trial of 50% oxygen via a Venturi mask is indicated. One can argue that hyperinflation therapy was not indicated. If the right lower lobe infiltrate was atelectatic, such therapy certainly would be indicated, and on a trial basis in this case, after the second assessment, such therapy provokes no quarrel.

The **last assessment** shows that vigorous therapy pays off. The patient appears to be improving nicely, and the infiltrate in the right lower lobe has disappeared. This strongly suggests that the cause of the infiltrate was postobstructive atelectasis and *not* pneumonia.

What was *not* included in the final assessment and plan was an injunction to assess the patient's knowledge of her respiratory hygiene program. Specifically, this assessment should include a review of her knowledge of the first signs of pulmonary infection and the methodology for any aerosol devices described. Certainly a review and instructions for herself and her caregivers in chest percussion and postural drainage techniques are in order. A review demonstration of appropriate use of the flutter valve also should be required.

Chapter 5   Asthma

Response 1

S: "I feel horrible, and my chest is tight."

O: Pursed-lip breathing; cyanotic appearance; use of accessory muscles of inspiration; frequent, strong cough productive of moderate amount of thick, white mucus; vital signs: BP 110/85, HR 190, RR 28, afebrile; bilateral diminished breath sounds, wheezing, and rhonchi; PEFR 150 lpm; CXR: air trapping and depressed diaphragm; SpO_2 (2 L/min O_2 by nasal cannula) 77%; ABGs: pH 7.45, $PaCO_2$ 28, HCO_3^- 19, PaO_2 40

A: • Status asthmaticus (general history and clinical data)
 • Increased work of breathing (HR, RR, and use of accessory muscles)
 • Bronchospasm (wheezing and PEFR)
 • Excessive bronchial secretions but effective cough (sputum production)
 • Acute alveolar hyperventilation and metabolic acidosis with severe hypoxemia (lactic acid probably causing pH and HCO_3^- to be lower than expected for an acute decrease in $PaCO_2$ level)
  Possible impending ventilatory failure

P: Up-regulate Oxygen Therapy Protocol (e.g., 4 lpm nasal cannula or HAFOE at FIO_2 40%). Begin aggressive Aerosolized Medication Protocol (e.g., albuterol aerosol per continuous medication/heliox nebulizer, at 20 mg/h). Initiate Bronchial Hygiene Therapy Protocol (e.g., C&DB q2h, bland aerosol therapy if tolerated, and prn suctioning). Maintain ventilator/intubation equipment on standby. Continue to monitor (e.g., vital signs, breath sounds, pulse oximetry, ABGs, and PEFR). Continue or increase frequency (6 puffs q8h) of beclomethasone inhaler as prescribed for home use.

Response 2

S: "I'm wheezing too much, and I can't go to sleep."

O: Pursed-lip breathing; cyanotic appearance; use of accessory muscles of inspiration; frequent, strong cough; moderate amount of thick, white mucus; PEFR 175 lpm; vital signs: BP 105/82, HR 180, RR 24; prolonged expiration; bilateral diminished breath sounds, wheezing, and rhonchi; SpO_2 95%; ABGs: pH 7.48, $PaCO_2$ 34, HCO_3^- 24, PaO_2 73

A: • Continued increased work of breathing (vital signs, use of accessory muscles, ABGs)
 • Bronchospasm (wheezing and PEFR)
 • Thick bronchial secretions (sputum production)
 • Acute alveolar hyperventilation with mild hypoxemia improving (metabolic acidosis corrected)
  Impending ventilatory failure still a possibility

P: Continue Oxygen Therapy, Bronchial Hygiene Therapy, and Aerosolized Medication Protocols. Continue beclomethasone inhaler as prescribed for home use. Maintain ventilator on standby. Continue to monitor and reevaluate closely.

Response 3

S: "I feel like there is a weight on my chest."

O: Use of accessory muscles; pursed-lip breathing; skin: damp, cool, and cyanotic; no cough or sputum; PEFR 145 lpm; vital signs: BP 160/100, HR 185, RR 13; diminished breath sounds bilaterally; no wheezing or rhonchi; SpO_2 79%; ABGs: pH 7.27, $PaCO_2$ 57, HCO_3^- 24, PaO_2 51

A: • Patient becoming fatigued (no wheezing, vital signs, ABGs)
    • Worsening bronchospasm ("silent chest," with decreased wheezing and decreased sputum production)
    • Acute ventilatory failure with moderate hypoxemia (ABGs)

P: Contact physician stat regarding ventilatory failure. Consider intubation and mechanical ventilation. Until then up-regulate Oxygen Therapy Protocol (e.g., nonrebreathing mask @ FIO_2 1.0). Continue Aerosolized Medication and Bronchial Hygiene Protocols. Continue beclomethasone inhaler as prescribed for home use. Monitor continuously. Request chest x-ray after intubation.

DISCUSSION

The historical point that the patient not only has asthma but also has had it severely enough recently to require hospitalizations and ventilator support is important and should alert the respiratory care practitioner that this patient is more than the run-of-the-mill asthmatic. That the patient's mother has stopped smoking, made environmental changes at home, and been faithful enough to have the child on a home-recording program of peak expiratory flow rates (PEFRs) and that the child has been desensitized speak to a compliant and intelligent patient and family.

The clinical manifestations presented in this case are all associated with **bronchospasm** (see Fig. 1-11) and **excessive bronchial secretions** (see Fig. 1-12). The pursed-lip breathing, cyanosis, prolonged expirations, use of accessory muscles of respiration, frequent cough, thick, white mucus, increased heart rate and blood pressure, and the severity of the child's hypoxemia (despite alveolar hyperventilation on admission) are all good severity indicators and suggest that vigorous therapy is necessary. Many respiratory specialists feel that sputum and blood eosinophilia are good markers for allergic exacerbations of asthma. A circulating eosinophil count or Wright's stain for sputum eosinophilia, or both, might have been in order.

Note in **Response 1** that the pH and HCO_3^- levels are lower than expected for a particular $PaCO_2$ level, most likely because of the *lactic acid* caused by the severe hypoxemia. The lactic acid offsets the increased pH and HCO_3^- levels that should develop immediately in response to an acutely decreased $PaCO_2$ level–according to the $PaCO_2/HCO_3/$-pH nomogram. (A $PaCO_2$ of 28 should move the pH to a level greater than 7.52.) The patient's arterial blood gas values (ABGs: pH 7.45, $PaCO_2$ 28, HCO_3^- 19, and PaO_2 40) are often interpreted *incorrectly* as *chronic alveolar hyperventilation with hypoxemia.*

In this case the following *two* primary indicators confirm that the patient has acute alveolar hyperventilation with hypoxemia and not chronic alveolar hyperventilation:

1. The patient's age and history of acute asthmatic episodes
2. The severe hypoxemia enough to cause slight anaerobic metabolism

Because of the increased work of breathing (vital signs) and acute alveolar hyperventilation, the possibility of impending ventilatory failure is real.

At this point, however, the child is not retaining carbon dioxide, so increasing the nasal oxygen therapy to 4 L/min or, alternatively, using a Venturi mask is reasonable. The child needs frequent bronchodilator and inhaled steroid therapy, which should have been started. The semicritical nature of her illness and impending ventilatory failure should have been reported to the physician immediately after the first assessment. Intravenous corticosteroid medications are used almost always in this setting. Increasingly, continuous nebulized bronchodilator therapy is used in children such as this girl.

The time of the **second assessment** is more than 2 hours into aggressive therapy. The patient is improving slightly. The physical findings have changed little, and she still demonstrates mild hypoxemia. Assuming that the patient's oxygen therapy was increased correctly after the first assessment, a key point to note is that hypoxemia is present despite oxygen therapy. Further increase in the oxygen therapy would be safe. Use of a nonrebreathing oxygen mask would be appropriate. Hydration of the patient (and her secretions) would be helpful, probably via the parenteral route. Close monitoring of vital signs, pulse oximetry, breath sounds, PEFR determinations, and judicious use of arterial or capillary sample blood gas analyses should continue.

By the time of the **final case scenario** (Response 3), the patient's status asthmaticus clearly has worsened to the point of acute ventilatory failure. Significant carbon dioxide retention and persistent severe hypoxemia are present. The silent chest does not represent improved bronchoconstriction. Rather, it suggests that a marked diminution of gas flow has occurred so that breath sounds are no longer generated. Confirmation comes from the fact that the patient can no longer cough up secretions. Presumably they too are being expectorated with difficulty, given the obstructed airway. A chest x-ray to rule out bilateral pneumothorax as a cause of the bilaterally diminished breath sounds is a good idea.

The therapist at this point should not leave the patient and should be prepared to bag and mask or (if allowed in the individual institution) to go ahead with emergency intubation. The patient's hypertension and tachycardia suggest that further administration of bronchodilator aerosol alone is contraindicated, unless or until the patient has a mechanically open airway.

KEY POINT ANSWERS

For Asthma (DRG* 98)

1. Basic Concept Formation
   a. *Yes.* True bronchial asthma, triggered by exposure to *extrinsic antigens,* commonly begins in childhood. It frequently is associated with other symptoms of allergy, such as *allergic rhinitis* (hay fever) or hives.
   b. *Yes,* although less commonly than children. In adults the asthma often is *not* related to extrinsic allergy, such as pollen, dust, and danders. Often it follows bouts of respiratory infection. It is called *intrinsic asthma,* or *asthmatic bronchitis.*
   c. *Yes.* The main pathophysiologic mechanisms activated in asthma are *airway inflammation and hyperreactivity,* resulting in mucus *hypersecretion and bronchoconstriction.*
   d. *Not necessarily.* The patient or caregiver is required to *assess and treat* the condition, much as the respiratory care practitioner practicing in the therapist-driven protocol (TDP) paradigm. Multiple therapeutic strategies and modalities often are required to achieve good "control" of the patient's symptoms. Even with optimal outpatient and home care, exacerbations of asthma may require patient visits to the emergency department or hospitalization.
   e. *No. Dyspnea and wheezing* are the most common symptoms of asthma.
   f. *Yes,* see answer 1.d. Such analysis and treatment selection by the patient or caregiver are the basis for the National Asthma Education Project (NAEP) guidelines.[†]
   g. Inhaled *antiallergic or antiinflammatory agents,* such as cromolyn sodium, nedocromil, or inhaled steroids and beta-agonist and anticholinergic bronchodilator aerosols are used. Avoidance of allergens and immunotherapy (desensitization injections) are other avenues of approach.
   h. As with pneumothorax, massive pulmonary embolism, and foreign body aspiration, asthma often presents fairly acute, with a *crisis onset* over a few minutes or hours. Symptoms may abate as quickly as they arise. Approximately 50% of asthmatic children seem to outgrow their asthma by the time of puberty. By adulthood, more than 75% of childhood asthmatics are improved greatly or no longer symptomatic.
2. Database Formation
   a. Inflammation
   b. Asthma is a chronic lung disease characterized by airway obstruction and narrowing (which may or may not be reversible), airway inflammation, and airway hyperresponsiveness to a variety of stimuli. Airway smooth muscle contraction and mucus hypersecretion that causes airway obstruction are the primary abnormalities in cases of asthma.[‡]
   c. The following commonly recognized *types* of asthma are classified by their triggers:
      1. Extrinsic asthma (see answer 1.b)
      2. Intrinsic asthma (asthmatic bronchitis) (see answer 1.b)
      3. Exercise-induced asthma

---

*DRG, *Diagnosis-related group.*
†NAEP: *Guidelines for the diagnosis and management of asthma, DHHS Expert Panel Report, 1991.*
‡See color plate 6 in Des Jardins T, Burton GG: *Clinical manifestations & assessment of respiratory disease, ed 4,* St. Louis, 2002, Mosby, Inc.

4. Cough-variant asthma
5. Cold-induced asthma
6. Fume- or vapor-induced asthma (reactive airway disease [RADS])
7. Catamenial (menses-related) asthma

d. *Increased airway resistance and decreased ventilation/perfusion ratio (shunt)* are the primary pathophysiologic mechanisms responsible for the *clinical manifestations* of asthma (see Fig. 1-7). *Air trapping, retained or excessive secretions,* and *chemoreceptor discharge* are secondary mechanisms.

e. The airway model (see Fig. 1-14) consists of airway wall, lumen, and supporting structures. The wall and lumen components are abnormal in asthmatics. Some investigators believe that the supporting structures, that is, the lung parenchyma, also may be abnormal in individuals with chronic asthma.

f. According to the NAEP guidelines, effective management of asthma, which can prevent exacerbations, relies on the following *four essential components,* each with separate goals:
1. Objective measures of lung function to *assess and monitor* the *severity* of the asthma exacerbation
2. Pharmacologic therapy to *relieve symptoms* by reducing airway inflammation
3. Environmental measures to *control allergens and irritants*
4. Patient education to *improve patient knowledge of the disease*
Patient education should include efforts to educate the patient's family. Parent, teacher, and community education is important for the proper diagnosis and management of asthma in pediatric and adolescent patients. *Good control* of asthma results in shorter, less frequent, and less severe exacerbations; fewer trips to the doctor's office or hospital; and longer symptom-free intervals between asthmatic attacks.

g. *Treatment* (TDP selection) as follows:
1. *Bronchial Hygiene Therapy Protocol* (see Fig. 1-12 and Protocol 1-2): For lumen obstruction, see airway model, Fig. 1-14. Perform deep breathing and coughing, suctioning, airway (bland aerosol) and systemic hydration, and occasionally therapeutic bronchoscopy.
2. *Aerosolized Medication Protocol* (see Fig. 1-11 and Protocol 1-4): For wall abnormalities, see airway model, Fig. 1-14. Administer aerosolized *antiinflammatory* agents (corticosteroids and nonsteroidal antiinflammatory agents, such as cromolyn and nedocromil) and, rarely, decongestants.
3. Perform *Oxygen Therapy Protocol* (see Protocol 1-1) as needed for hypoxemia.

Modality	Typical Therapies Ordered	Expected Outcomes	Monitors
Oxygen therapy (see Protocol 1-1)	Oxygen per nasal cannula 4 L/min	Increased PaO_2, SpO_2; normalizing $PaCO_2$, heart rate, respiratory rate	$SpO_2 \geq 92\%$; ECG
Aerosolized medication therapy (see Protocol 1-4)	Albuterol 0.2 ml in 2 ml normal saline q30min × 3	Less dyspnea; less wheezing; improved ease of expectoration	$SpO_2 \geq 92\%$; improved PEFR
Antiinflammatory aerosol therapy	Beclomethasone 4 puffs q2h × 4	See previous modality	See previous modality
Bronchial hygiene therapy (Protocol 1-2)	Postural drainage, chest physical therapy, cough and deep breaths q4h	See aerosolized medication therapy	See aerosolized medication therapy; increased sputum production

Continued

3. Assessment
   a. *Yes.* The symptoms of an acute asthma exacerbation included episodic, worsening *dyspnea* and (to a lesser extent) *cough* productive of thick, tenacious sputum. The signs of asthma, that is its *clinical manifestations,* include her falling PEFR, her appearance ("tripod" stance, pursed-lip breathing, barrel chest deformity, use of accessory muscles, and cyanosis), rapid heart and respiratory rate, findings on chest auscultation (wheezes and rhonchi), and laboratory findings (hyperinflation on chest x-ray, hypoxemia in ABGs, and obstructive physiology demonstration on pulmonary function tests [PFTs]).
   b. *Yes.* The initial signs and symptoms in this case, especially when taken with the history, are practically pathognomonic of the pathophysiologic mechanisms seen in asthma (see Fig. 1-11). The clinical manifestations of asthma are as follows:
      1. Falling PEFR; wheezes suggesting *increased airway resistance*
      2. Appearance (tripod stance, pursed-lip breathing, barrel chest, use of accessory muscles) suggesting *increased work of breathing*
      3. Cyanosis and hypoxemia on ABGs reflecting *shunt physiology*
      4. Rapid heart rate, labored, rapid breathing, and chest tightness suggesting *cardiopulmonary distress* and *hypoxemia*
      5. Diminished breath sounds, wheezing, rhonchi, and air trapping on admission chest x-ray suggesting *increased airway resistance and alveolar hyperinflation*
   c. The *initial indications of severity* in this case include impending ventilatory failure, severe breathlessness, cough, chest tightness, wheezing in a relatively silent chest, tachycardia, tachypnea, use of accessory muscles, cyanosis, and profound hypoxemia on supplemental oxygen despite alveolar hyperventilation.
4. Application
   a. Oxygen therapy *was* indicated because of the patient's severe hypoxemia.
   b. Monitoring of heart rate, rhythm, electrocardiogram (ECG) morphology, ABGs and pulse oximetry *was* indicated because of the patient's severe respiratory distress, tachycardia, and hypoxemia.
   c. Bronchial hygiene therapy *was* indicated because of the need for mucolysis and expectoration to clear mucus in the obstructed airways. Postural drainage and chest percussion *may have been tried* to aid in expectoration of thick, tenacious secretions. This modality is often not tolerated during severe asthmatic exacerbations.
   d. Aerosolized medication therapy *was* indicated because of the diagnosis of *bronchial asthma* with wheezing.
   e. Hyperinflation therapy *was not* indicated because the patient had no evidence of atelectasis and already demonstrated air trapping.
   f. Intubation and mechanical ventilation *were not* indicated because the other therapies (see answers 4.a to 4.d) had not yet been tried and the patient was under close observation.
5. Evaluation
   a. See answer 2.h.
   b. See answer 2.h.
   c. Limits of suggested therapies, as follows:
      1. *Bronchial hygiene therapy:* Bland aerosol therapy is not tolerated at all by many asthmatics, and mucolytics such as acetylcysteine are relatively contraindicated because of their tendency to cause or worsen airway inflammation and to cause bronchospasm. Suctioning may be done as frequently

as tolerated (as much as every 2 to 3 minutes), and percussion and postural drainage (PD) are generally not tolerated well at all. Therapeutic bronchoscopy may be done as frequently as new, otherwise untreatable atelectasis develops distal to obstructive airways.

2. *Aerosolized medication therapy:* This therapy may be given (under close monitoring of heart rate) *continuously* in cases of status asthmaticus. Antiinflammatory therapy may be given initially via MDI aerosol every hour, then every 3 to 4 hours.

3. *Oxygen therapy:* The upper limit of nasal cannula oxygen therapy is 5 to 6 L/min; mask F_{IO_2} may be increased to 1 as determined by repeat ABG analysis and is limited by CO_2 retention.

d. *Advantages of treatment modalities:* All are relatively inexpensive (except bronchoscopy) and, with the monitors outlined in answer 2.h, relatively safe. The most cost-effective approach over the long term is *prevention of exacerbations,* which appears to have been attempted in this patient right along. If because of the patient's metabolic acidosis the reader has elected *initially* to intubate and *mechanically ventilate* the patient, the benefits and adverse effects of that modality (e.g., barotrauma) should be reviewed.

e. If the patient *improves,* first reduce the F_{IO_2} and frequency of aerosolized bronchodilator treatments. Wait 24 to 48 hours before greatly reducing the frequency of administration of the aerosolized steroids to less than every 4 to 6 hours.

f. If *little improvement* occurs with oxygen, bronchial hygiene, and bronchodilator and antiinflammatory aerosol therapy, do not hesitate to quickly intubate and mechanically ventilate this patient. If atelectasis were present, bronchoscopy and intubation would be done at the same sitting.

6. Boundary Awareness

a. At the time of the *second* assessment the following parameters had worsened or not significantly improved: heart rate and apparent *persistent increased work of breathing.* Her ABGs looked better, although to know this for sure, calculation of the A-a oxygen gradient is necessary.

b. *Yes.* The patient can be shown how to assess her own symptoms and peak flow rates. The caregiver can be instructed in assessment of the severity of her daughter's symptoms and in the use of new modalities if applicable.

c. A supervisor probably should have been asked for help at the time of the *first* assessment. Children with status asthmaticus are virtually never "no code," and aggressive care generally is required by all concerned. This child is acutely ill, in impending ventilatory failure, and probably will be transferred to an intensive care unit (ICU). Certainly a supervisor should have been consulted by the time of the *third* assessment, when acute ventilatory failure had occurred.

d. Depending on personal preference in such cases, certainly the physician should have been called by the time of the *third* assessment. In fact, most respiratory care protocols state that the physician should be notified when ventilatory failure is impending.

e. *Ventilatory failure* is diagnosed on the basis of resistant hypoxemia and progressive carbon dioxide retention with acidemia.

f. Severe asthma, which is episodic by definition, may progress to continuous asthma, which is called *status asthmaticus.* Unless this condition is terminated quickly, ventilatory failure will develop. Spontaneous pneumothorax may complicate asthma, or it may be a result of ventilator-induced *barotrauma.* Hypercorticism secondary to corticosteroid therapy also may occur, although not usually as a result of *aerosolized* steroid therapy. *Tachycardia* and *cardiac arrhythmias* may result from excessive beta-stimulant bronchodilator therapy.

Chapter 6   *Pneumonia*

Response 1

S: Patient states that he is very short of breath and has had a nonproductive cough for the last 4 days.

O: Vital signs: BP 165/90, HR 120, RR 33, T 39.5° C (103° F); cough: frequent, strong, hacking, productive of small amount of white and yellow sputum; skin: pale and damp; over right lower lobe, increased tactile and vocal fremitus, dull percussion note, bronchial breath sounds; SpO_2 87%; ABGs (on 2 L/min O_2 nasal cannula): pH 7.56, $PaCO_2$ 24, HCO_3^- 22, PaO_2 56; CXR: right lower lung infiltrate, air bronchograms, and alveolar consolidation; WBC 21,000/mm^3

A: • Respiratory distress (vital signs, ABGs)
 • Right lower lobe pneumonia: consolidation (fever, fremitus, percussion notes, bronchial breath sounds, and CXR)
 • Bronchial secretions: infection likely (white and yellow sputum)
     Good ability to mobilize bronchial secretions (strong cough)
 • Acute alveolar hyperventilation with mild hypoxemia (ABGs)

P: Initiate Oxygen Therapy Protocol (e.g., increasing from 2 to 4 lpm per nasal cannula). Bronchial Hygiene Therapy Protocol (e.g., C&DB 2×/shift). Obtain sputum for Gram stain and culture; induce if necessary. Begin trial period of Hyperinflation Therapy Protocol (e.g., incentive spirometry 2×/shift). Monitor and reevaluate.

Response 2

S: "I feel worse than when I came in."

O: Vital signs: BP 140/70, HR 125, RR 35 and shallow, T 38.9° C (102° F); strong, barking cough; producing small amount of blood-streaked sputum; cyanosis; over right lower and middle lung lobes and left lower lobe, increased tactile and vocal fremitus, dull percussion notes, bronchial breath sounds, and crackles; SpO_2 86%; ABGs: pH 7.55, $PaCO_2$ 26, HCO_3^- 24, PaO_2 53

A: • Continued respiratory distress (vital signs, ABGs)
 • Alveolar consolidation or atelectasis likely in right lower and middle lobes and left lower lobe; condition possibly worsening (percussion notes and breath sounds, crackles)
 • Bronchial secretions: small amount (sputum production)
 • Acute alveolar hyperventilation with moderate hypoxemia; essentially unchanged (ABGs)

P: Update physician on patient's respiratory status. Continue Bronchial Hygiene Therapy Protocol. Continue trial period of Hyperinflation Therapy Protocol. Up-regulate Oxygen Therapy Protocol (e.g., simple oxygen mask or partial rebreathing oxygen mask @ FIO_2 = 0.50). Ensure that patient is sitting up when taking oral medications, food, and liquids. Continue to monitor and reevaluate.

Response 3

S: "I'm breathing easier."

O: Vital signs: BP 135/85, HR 90, RR 19, T 37.3° C (99° F); cough: strong and nonproductive; CXR: resolving pneumonia, consolidation or atelectasis in lower and middle right and lower left lobes; increased tactile and vocal fremitus, dull percussion notes, and bronchial breath sounds; SpO_2 97%; ABGs: pH 7.44, $PaCO_2$ 35, HCO_3^- 24, PaO_2 163

A: • Consolidation or atelectasis in right lower and middle and left lower lobes—resolving (CXR, chest assessment data)
  • Normal acid-base status with overly corrected hypoxemia (ABGs)

P: Down-regulate Hyperinflation Therapy Protocol (e.g., reducing incentive spirometry to 1×/shift with supervision, plus patient instruction). Continue to encourage C&DB. Down-regulate oxygen therapy per protocol (e.g., 3 lpm nasal cannula). Check final results of sputum culture. Reevaluate next shift.

DISCUSSION

This patient has a typical case of pneumonia, with cough, fever, increased blood pressure, heart rate and respiratory rate, dull percussion note, bronchial breath sounds, chest x-ray infiltrates, and acute alveolar hyperventilation with hypoxemia (see **pneumonic consolidation,** Fig. 1-9). Initially the respiratory therapist's attention should be directed to identifying the causative agent by inducing a sputum specimen for culture and to oxygenating the patient, in this case with a low-flow oxygen cannula.

Unfortunately no effective, specific respiratory care treatment modality exists for alveolar consolidation. Hyperinflation therapy may be beneficial, especially when applied to partially consolidated alveoli. Just like any treatment modality, however, the effectiveness of the hyperinflation therapy must be assessed through the collection of objective data (e.g., arterial blood gases, chest x-ray, or vital signs). In addition, the response to oxygen therapy is often poor because the patient almost certainly has a right-to-left intrapulmonary shunt across the pneumonic segment. Some ventilated and perfused alveoli hopefully can pick up some of the deficit, but a degree of oxygen refractoriness should be expected when alveolar consolidation is present.

This patient is so hypoxemic, despite alveolar hyperventilation, that close monitoring obviously is necessary. Asking questions about the patient's alcoholism and pneumonia vaccine status are worthwhile and show that the therapist is thinking beyond the immediate acute episode during the evaluation and treatment of the patient.

The **second assessment** reflects that patients with pneumonia often feel worse when in fact they are improving. The production of sputum often is seen as a worrisome event when actually it may herald the breaking up of the pneumonic infiltrate. Because the patient is still producing some sputum, bronchial hygiene therapy should be continued. The patient's PaO_2 really has not improved significantly, and a trial of a higher concentration of oxygen by Venturi or nonrebreathing oxygen mask may be helpful at this point. Improved oxygenation would help allay the patient's anxiety, as well as that of the physician and treating therapist.

The **third assessment** shows that the patient clearly is improving. Down-regulation of the oxygen therapy toward room air is all that remains for the therapist to do. Ordinarily hyperinflation therapy would be reduced or discontinued in preparation for an early discharge. The reader should recognize that the average length of stay for patients with pneumonia in an American hospital today is approximately 4 days. Such patients leave the hospital with a resolving, but not completely cleared, pneumonic process (and x-ray). Improvement in the patient's clinical status and resolution of fever, dyspnea, and signs of toxicity, however, can and should be expected in this short period unless complications such as bacteremia, abscess, or empyema arise. Attention to the event that precipitated the admission is worthwhile, and review of the situation and recollection that this patient is a problem drinker would be appropriate before discharge, when attempts to interdict this problem might be most helpful.

KEY POINT ANSWERS

For Pneumonia (DRG* 78, 89, 90)

1. Basic Concept Formation
   a. *No.* It is usually caused by an acute exposure to a sometimes contagious infectious agent. Identification of the precise causative infectious agent is helpful because it allows for specific (targeted) antibiotic therapy.
   b. *Yes.* The cough is not always productive, and obtaining a sputum specimen (see answer 1.a) is one of the *first tasks* of the respiratory care practitioner (RCP) dealing with this condition.
   c. *Antibiotics* are used in *all* bacterial pneumonias and in a few viral pneumonias.
   d. *Yes.* In the United States, pneumonia is the sixth leading cause of death and the number one cause of death from infectious disease. One fifth of the estimated 4 million U.S. cases per year require hospitalization. The overall mortality of community acquired pneumonia (CAP) is 1% to 5%, but it may reach 25% in certain segments of the population (see answers 2.b).
2. Database Formation
   a. Pneumonia usually is an acute disease characterized by alveolar filling, called *consolidation,* in the case of most bacterial pneumonias† and by *interstitial infiltration and thickening* in many viral pneumonias.
   b. Different bacteria and viruses are *responsible* for pneumonia in different segments of the population, as follows:
      1. Chronic obstructive pulmonary disease (COPD) patients: *Streptococcus pneumoniae, Haemophilus influenzae,* and *Moraxella catarrhalis* (previously known as *Branhamella catarrhalis*)
      2. Cystic fibrosis patients: *Pseudomonas* and staphylococci
      3. Viral pneumonia patients: Prone to bacterial superinfection with *S. pneumoniae, H. influenzae,* and *Staphylococcus aureus.*
      4. Nursing home patients: Methicillin-resistant *S. aureus, Mycobacterium tuberculosis,* gram-negative bacilli, respiratory syncytial virus (RSV), adenovirus, and influenza virus
      5. Alcoholics: Aspiration pneumonia caused by oral or gastrointestinal flora (often with anaerobic organisms)
      6. Intubated patients and patients with neurologic disorders, e.g., post-cerebrovascular accident (CVA): aspiration pneumonia
   c. The *main pathophysiologic mechanisms* activated by infectious alveolar consolidation (pneumonia) are the *immune response, shunt physiology, and decreased lung compliance* (see Fig. 1-9). In cases of acute interstitial pneumonia, *alveolar-capillary diffusion block* is present, and the lung demonstrates stiffness or reduced compliance (see Fig. 1-10).
   d. *Severe* CAP is defined by the presence of one or more of the following clinical findings:
      1. Respiratory frequency >30 breaths per minute
      2. PaO_2/FiO_2 ratio <25 mm Hg
      3. Requirement of mechanical ventilation
      4. Involvement of multiple lobes or an increase in the size of the opacity by 50%

---

†See color plate 7 in Des Jardins T, Burton GG: *Clinical manifestations and assessment of respiratory disease, ed 4,* St. Louis, 2002, Mosby.

KEY POINT ANSWERS—cont'd

     5. Shock: systolic BP <90 mm Hg, diastolic BP <60 mm Hg
     6. Vasopressor required for more than 4 hours
     7. Urine output <20 ml/h, or <50 ml/4 h
     8. Acute renal failure requiring dialysis

  e. Criteria for consideration of *hospitalization* of CAP patients include the following:
     1. Respiratory distress
     2. High fever
     3. Hypotension (systolic BP <100)
     4. Altered mental status
     5. Suppurative or metastatic infection
     6. Significant coexisting disease
     7. Severe laboratory abnormalities (that is, metabolic acidosis, elevated BUN and serum creatinine levels, hypernatremia >155 mmol/L)

  f. The *goals of therapy* in individuals with pneumonia, along with use of appropriate systemic antibiotics, are as follows:
     1. Prevention (with pneumococcal or influenza vaccine) when appropriate
     2. Fever control
     3. Dyspnea control
     4. Relief of hypoxemia
     5. Clearance of airway secretions if present
     6. Ventilatory support if necessary

  g. *Oxygen Therapy Protocol* (see Protocol 1-1) in all hypoxemic patients: *Bronchial Hygiene Therapy Protocol* in patients with excessive, poorly mobilized secretions (in the resolution phase of pneumonia); *ventilatory support* in the presence of acute ventilatory failure

  h. *Empyema, pleural effusion, involvement of other lobes, septicemia,* and *ventilatory failure* are complications of pneumonia.

3. Assessment
  a. *Yes.* The patient reported fever, chills, and cough. He demonstrated respiratory distress, tachycardia, physical and x-ray findings indicating alveolar consolidation, and oxygen-resistant hypoxemia despite alveolar hyperventilation.

  b. *Yes.* His *reduced ventilation-perfusion ratio* and *relative shunt physiology were evidenced in oxygen-refractory hypoxemia.* His alveolar consolidation resulted in *decreased lung compliance,* evidenced on chest physical examination by shallow, rapid breathing, and findings of alveolar consolidation on the admission chest x-ray film. His *immune response* was evidenced by his fever and elevated white blood cell count.

  c. Initially, only his *respiratory rate* of 33/min indicated the severity. At the *second assessment* the pneumonic process apparent in *additional lobes* reflected the condition's worsening severity.

4. Application
  a. Sputum sample/induction *was* indicated because the patient was expectorating yellowish sputum. If the RCP did not think to "catch" some sputum when it was available, he or she *could* elect to induce it.

  b. Oxygen therapy *was* indicated to try to relieve the patient's modest but real hypoxemia.

  c. Bronchial hygiene initially *was* indicated because the patient had some secretions. Encouragement of cough and deep breathing initially was appropriate. Failure to recognize this step costs American hospitals millions of dollars each year.

d. Aerosolized medication therapy *was not* indicated because pneumonia is primarily an anatomic alteration of the alveoli.

e. Hyperinflation therapy *was* indicated because of evidence of atelectasis (pulmonary infiltrate). For example, a trial of incentive spirometry to prevent or treat any coincident atelectasis *may* have been appropriate. The therapeutic effect of hyperinflation therapy for consolidation is often disappointing. However, a trial period may be worth the effort.

5. Evaluation

a. The following results are to be expected:

1. *Sputum induction:* expect to induce a satisfactory sputum sample promptly.

2. *Oxygen therapy:* expect to modestly, but not totally, improve the patient's hypoxemia. The degree of success is inversely proportional to the degree of absolute shunt present. Improving the patient's hypoxemia may improve his dyspnea.

3. *Bronchial hygiene:* expect to loosen secretions and keep airways clear. This therapy also works to prevent mucus plugging and atelectasis.

4. *Hyperinflation therapy:* expect to offset the development of atelectasis and improve oxygenation.

b. *Pulse oximetry* would be helpful to monitor the patient's hypoxemia. Follow-up ABGs and chest x-ray films are appropriate.

c. *Oxygen therapy* can be increased to an FIO_2 of 1.0. If this action is not sufficient, the patient could be intubated and placed on an FIO_2 of 0.8 to 1.0, and a peak end-expiratory pressure (PEEP) trial attempted. Severe pneumonia may improve with this approach, but it was not indicated here.

d. Consider *intubation* as in answer 5.c.

6. Boundary Awareness

a. *Pulse oximetry and ABG analysis* are the best means to assess improvement. *Lysis of fever* often signals improvement; *persistent fever* is a sign of inappropriate initial antibiotic selection; *recurrent fever* is often a sign of bacterial or viral superinfection. An initial worsening of the chest x-ray film after patient hydration has been achieved and parenteral antibiotics given is not unusual. However, in cases of severe CAP, extension of the infiltrate on the chest x-ray film may be an ominous sign.

b. *No,* not necessarily, if you are comfortable with the patient's lack of severity indicators.

c. You probably should not call the physician at all. The patient demonstrated continued improvement in fever and ABGs by the time of the *third assessment.*

d. *Ventilatory failure* was never an issue because his $PaCO_2$ was never elevated and his PaO_2 was stable or improving.

Chapter 7   Human Immunodeficiency Virus (HIV)

Response 1

S: Sore throat and extremely irritating, nonproductive cough

O: Cough: frequent, strong, and nonproductive; neck: swollen lymph nodes; vital signs: BP 137/90, HR 95, RR 20, T 37° C (98.6° F); lung bases: dull percussion notes and bronchial breath sounds; CXR: infiltrates in lung bases (possible pneumonia); ABGs (room air): pH 7.47, $Paco_2$ 33, HCO_3^- 23, Pao_2 76; WBC 7500/mm^3

A: • Increased work of breathing (general appearance, vital signs, ABGs)
    • Alveolar consolidation (pneumonia) in lung bases (CXR, bronchial breath sounds, dull percussion notes)
    • Acute alveolar hyperventilation with mild hypoxemia (ABGs)

P: Initiate continuous pulse oximetry, set to alarm at Spo_2 <90%. As per Oxygen Therapy Protocol, administer 2 lpm by nasal cannula. C&DB 2×/shift per Hyperinflation Therapy Protocol. Use incentive spirometer; instruct and leave at bedside. Induce sputum for Gram stain and culture. Monitor and reevaluate every shift.

Response 2

S: "I'm not breathing very well. I'm getting worse."

O: Cough: frequent, strong, and nonproductive; vital signs: BP 185/100, HR 125, RR 31, rectal T 37° C (98.6° F); RML, RLL, and LLL: dull percussion notes and bronchial breath sounds; Spo_2 92%; ABGs: pH 7.54, $Paco_2$ 27, HCO_3^- 22, Pao_2 54.

A: • Continued increased work of breathing (general appearance, vital signs, ABGs)
    • Alveolar consolidation in lung bases (earlier CXR and present bronchial breath sounds, dull percussion notes)
    • Acute alveolar hyperventilation with worsening hypoxemia (ABGs)
      Possible impending ventilatory failure

P: Up-regulate oxygen therapy by protocol: O_2 by 50% nonrebreather mask. Continue Hyperinflation Therapy Protocol. Contact physician regarding patient's tachypnea and worsening A-a O_2 gradient. Obtain repeat chest x-ray. Prepare for bronchoscopy/BAL if physician requests it. Consider transfer to ICU. Monitor and evaluate q2h.

Response 3

S: The patient made a head gesture that he was doing poorly.

O: No cough noted; vital signs: BP 170/85, HR 145, RR 30 and shallow, rectal T 40° C (104° F); dull percussion notes and bronchial breath sounds over RML, RLL, and LLL; CXR: greater density and air bronchograms: RML, RLL, and LLL; SpO_2 77%; ABGs: pH 7.28, $PaCO_2$ 61, HCO_3^- 27, PaO_2 47; WBC 15,200/mm^3

A: • Continued increased work of breathing (general appearance, vital signs, ABGs)
   • Alveolar consolidation in RML, RLL, LLL worsening (CXR, bronchial breath sounds, dull percussion notes)
   • Acute ventilatory failure with severe hypoxemia (ABGs)

P: Contact physician stat: Consider mechanical ventilation, transfer to intensive care unit (ICU), and perform bronchoscopy. Up-regulate Oxygen Therapy Protocol (e.g., to FiO_2 = 1.0). Up-regulate Hyperinflation Therapy Protocol (e.g., trial of CPAP mask at 10 cm H_2O until decision about mechanical ventilation is made). Monitor and reevaluate.

DISCUSSION

This patient has an undiagnosed pulmonary infiltrate of uncertain duration. A history of irritating cough in an intravenous drug user and a pneumonic infiltrate on chest x-ray film should raise all sorts of red flags with the medical team. In this case it clearly did not. **On admission** his blood gases were not severely abnormal, although they showed mild resting hypoxemia despite alveolar hyperventilation. He apparently was admitted largely on the basis of the chest x-ray. At this point many clinicians would have elected to simply treat him as an outpatient with antibiotics and follow him in the clinic or office.

After the patient was admitted, he rapidly progressed to acute ventilatory failure with severe hypoxemia over the next 4 days. His chest x-ray and blood gases became worse, his dyspnea became more severe, and he became acutely febrile.

Note that 3 days into his hospitalization a diagnostic/therapeutic bronchoscopy was suggested in **Response 2**, basically because no *cause* for the pneumonia had been demonstrated. Also note that on the second assessment the patient's blood gases were significantly abnormal. Specifically, his PaO_2 had fallen from 76 to 54 mm Hg, despite the second blood gas being obtained, presumably, on a higher FiO_2 (the increase being assumed from Response 1). Calculation shows an enormous difference in the probable alveolar-arterial oxygen gradient between these two blood gases. The plan developed on the second evaluation suggests again that the treating therapist can do very little for pneumonia per se. Basically the therapist can attempt to oxygenate the patient, control airway secretions, and ensure (to the best ability) that the cause of the pneumonia is identified.

On the **final evaluation** the medical team becomes concerned that the patient may have acquired immunodeficiency syndrome (AIDS), and they order appropriate blood work. The therapist knows that respiratory treatment focuses on the *complications* of that syndrome, specifically the hypoxia and atelectasis associated with the **pneumonic consolidation** (see Fig. 1-9). The therapist must help ensure that appropriate biopsies and cultures are sent off once a bronchoscopy is performed (after the patient is on a ventilator). Because about 80% of acute, progressive pneumonias in patients testing positive for the human immunodeficiency virus (HIV) are caused by *Pneumocystis carinii* pneumonia (PCP), the therapist should ensure that special stains (Giemsa and silver methenamine) for PCP are performed in a timely manner.

Finally, in the last evaluation the reader should be aware that the patient has severe shunt physiology (severe refractory hypoxemia despite supplemental oxygen therapy) and acute ventilatory failure. The hypoxemia alone is enough to suggest to the therapist that the patient is approaching dangerous boundaries and that a stat call to the attending physician is indicated. In the last evaluation, intubation, ventilatory support, and positive end-expiratory pressure (PEEP) are almost certainly mandatory unless a "no-code" order is in effect per the patient's wishes.

Chapter 8   Lung Abscess

Response 1

S: "I spit all the time."

O: Thin, undernourished woman with poor hygiene; cyanotic appearance; frequent moderate-to-weak cough with foul-smelling, purulent sputum; vital signs: BP 145/75, HR 110, RR 33, T 39.3° C (102.8° F); right middle and upper lobes: tactile and vocal fremitus, crackles and rhonchi; ABGs (2 L/min by nasal cannula): pH 7.49, $PaCO_2$ 30, HCO_3^- 22, PaO_2 63; CXR: partially fluid-filled, 10-cm cavity in RUL and increased opacity in RML and RUL

A: • Increased work of breathing (general appearance, vital signs, ABGs)
  • Malnourished (inspection)
  • Lung abscess (RUL)–likely open to bronchus (CXR, sputum)
  • Consolidation versus atelectasis likely in RML and RUL (CXR: increased opacity)
  • Excessive bronchial secretions (purulent sputum)
      Moderate-to-weak cough
  • Acute alveolar hyperventilation with mild-to-moderate hypoxemia

P: Initiate Oxygen Therapy Protocol (e.g., 3 lpm per O_2 nasal cannula). Start Aerosolized Medication and Bronchial Hygiene Therapy Protocols (e.g., C&DB, PD to RUL and RML q4h; also, med. neb. with 2 cc 20% acetylcysteine with 0.5 cc albuterol qid). Obtain sputum for culture (i.e., aerobic, anaerobic, acid-fast, and fungal organisms) and sensitivity. Begin Hyperinflation Therapy Protocol (e.g., incentive spirometry qid and prn). Monitor closely (e.g., SpO_2 spot check in 1 hour, ABG in AM). Discuss need for social services and nutrition consults with attending physician.

Response 2

S: "I'm not as short of breath as I was yesterday."

O: Patient alert and oriented and no longer cyanotic; frequent and weak cough; sputum: thick and purulent; vital signs: BP 135/80, HR 98, RR 20, T 37.9° C (100.2° F); RML and RUL tactile and vocal fremitus, crackles, and rhonchi; ABGs: pH 7.48, $PaCO_2$ 34, HCO_3^- 23, PaO_2 81; SpO_2 96%

A: • Continued but improved respiratory distress (history)
  • Abscess (RUL) likely open to bronchus (CXR, sputum)
  • Consolidation or atelectasis likely in RUL and RML (CXR: increased opacity)
  • Excessive bronchial secretions (thick and purulent sputum)
  • Poor ability to mobilize secretions (weak cough)
  • Acute alveolar hyperventilation with corrected hypoxemia (ABGs)

P: Continue Oxygen Therapy, Aerosolized Medication, Bronchial Hygiene Therapy, and Hyperinflation Therapy Protocols. Monitor and reevaluate every shift.

Response 3

S: "You doctors cured my d...cough!"

O: Skin: normal color; no spontaneous cough; ability to produce a strong cough on request; no sputum noted; vital signs: BP 127/82, HR 86, RR 16, T 38° C (98.2° F); crackles over RLL; ABGs: pH 7.43, $PaCO_2$ 36, HCO_3^- 24, PaO_2 163; SpO_2 97%

A: • Abscess (RUL): improved (CXR, no sputum)
   • Consolidation and atelectasis still likely in RUL and RML (CXR: persistent infiltrate)
   • Normal acid-base status with overly corrected hypoxemia (ABGs)

P: Discontinue Oxygen Therapy, Bronchial Hygiene Therapy, and Hyperinflation Therapy Protocols. Discuss with physician patient training on MDIs (e.g., albuterol, 2 puffs qid and ipratropium 2 puffs qid). Also discuss patient training on C&DB and smoking cessation.

DISCUSSION

Production of foul-smelling, putrid, yellow-green sputum should immediately raise at least three diagnostic possibilities in the mind of the respiratory care practitioner: lung abscess, bronchiectasis, or communicating empyema (bronchopleural fistula). Several clinical manifestations presented in this case are associated directly with **excessive bronchial secretions** (see Fig. 1-12). For example, the patient had a productive cough, crackles, and rhonchi. That the patient has carious teeth and a vagrant lifestyle should be enough to make the diagnosis of lung abscess almost without a chest x-ray. At any rate, the patient clearly is acutely ill and febrile on arrival at the hospital. She has localized findings in the right lung, is moderately hypoxemic despite alveolar hyperventilation, and is chronically malnourished.

The **initial plan** to oxygenate, institute bronchial hygiene therapy, and suggest nutrition evaluation is entirely appropriate. Because the patient has had a clear change in mentation and is now confused, a toxic drug and alcohol blood screen is an excellent idea. A brain abscess, not uncommon in settings such as this, also should have been in the differential diagnosis. The patient's course within the next few days depends largely on clear mentation so that she can cooperate with the chest physical therapy procedures. To miss a toxic drug level of barbiturates, cocaine, or other sedatives would be tragic. The patient's alcohol consumption history speaks for itself. Finally, the possibility of a head injury (due to street lifestyle) cannot be ruled out. The reader who noted the confusion of the patient and said so in the subjective or objective analysis is to be congratulated.

The benefit of hyperinflation therapy may be marginal in this case. Infiltrates coincident with a lung cavity are almost certainly pneumonic. **Pneumonic consolidation** may not respond at all to lung expansion therapy (see Fig. 1-9). However, because **atelectasis** was also a possibility, a trial period of hyperinflation therapy was certainly warranted in this case (see Fig. 1-8).

At the time of the **second assessment** the patient's oxygenation is clearly being well served by her current oxygen and bronchial hygiene therapy. This is the time to check the laboratory to see whether sputum and blood cultures have been productive, in which case antibiotic therapy would need to be continued or regulated appropriately. In patients with infectious lung disease, the therapist should have this information available for the treating physician as soon as possible.

The **final assessment** indicates that the patient clearly has improved. This observation is correctly reflected in the therapist's assessment notes. The sequence of events necessitating this admission probably could be prevented in the future. The patient is asked to assume responsibility for continued improvement (e.g., smoking cessation, nutrition, clinic follow-ups, self-dosed MDI therapy, C&DB). Approximately 3 months later, the patient is doing well. A follow-up chest x-ray shows chronic scarring but no cavity in the right upper lobe.

Chapter 9 **Tuberculosis**

Response 1

S: "I can't get my breath."

O: Cyanosis, malnourishment, weakness, and obvious respiratory distress; cough: frequent, moderate amount of yellow sputum mixed with fresh blood, history of previous expectoration of blood; vital signs: BP 170/95, HR 110, RR 26, T 38.3° C (101° F); dull percussion notes, increased tactile and vocal fremitus, and bronchial breath sounds over the right and left lung bases; crackles and rhonchi in RUL; pleural friction rub: RLL between the 5th and 6th ribs in the anterior axillary line; CXR: LLL, RML, and RUL, increased opacity consistent with pneumonia; 5-cm cavity in LUL; ABGs (room air): pH 7.53, $PaCO_2$ 51, HCO_3^- 41, PaO_2 50; COHb 8.5 vol%; SpO_2 88%; WBC 14,000/mm^3

A: • Respiratory distress (general appearance, vital signs, ABGs)
  • Alveolar consolidation and atelectasis: LLL, RML, RUL (dull percussion notes, bronchial breath sounds, CXR)
  • Excessive bronchial secretions and hemoptysis (sputum production, rhonchi)
    Infection likely (yellow sputum)
    Effective cough (strong)
    Cavity LUL (CXR): probably tuberculous
  • Acute alveolar hyperventilation superimposed on chronic ventilatory failure with moderate hypoxemia (history, ABGs, CXR)
  • SpO_2 misleading because of COHb
  • Impending ventilatory failure

P: Initiate Oxygen Therapy Protocol (e.g., 2 lpm per nasal cannula). Check ABGs in 1 hour. Begin Bronchial Hygiene Therapy Protocol (e.g., C&DB, PD to posterior left upper chest 2×/shift). Obtain sputum for routine examination and AFB smear and culture 3 times. Start Hyperinflation Therapy Protocol (e.g., incentive spirometry qid). Monitor and reevaluate.

Response 2

S: "My cough is a lot better."

O: Improved cyanosis and respiratory distress; cough: frequent and productive of small amount of opaque sputum; vital signs: BP 143/90, HR 92, RR 18, T 37.4° C (99.3° F); dull percussion notes and bronchial breath sounds over lung bases; rhonchi over RML, but not as intense as on admission; positive tuberculin reaction; PFT: moderate-to-severe restrictive disorder; CXR: improved infiltrates on lung bases; ABGs: pH 7.48, $PaCO_2$ 60, HCO_3^- 42, PaO_2 61; SpO_2 91%

Response 2–cont'd

A: • Continued respiratory distress, but improving (vital signs, ABGs)
• Tuberculosis (positive tuberculin reaction, AFB smear)
• Alveolar consolidation or atelectasis, improving (history, CXR dull percussion notes, bronchial breath sounds)
• Excessive bronchial secretions in RML, improving (rhonchi)
• Acute alveolar hyperventilation superimposed on chronic ventilatory failure with mild hypoxemia, improving (ABGs)

P: Ensure respiratory isolation. Continue or up-regulate Oxygen Therapy Protocol (e.g., 3 lpm per nasal cannula and careful not to overoxygenate). Check ABGs in 1 hour. Continue Bronchial Hygiene Therapy Protocol. Continue or down-regulate Hyperinflation Therapy Protocol.

Response 3

S: "I'm ready to run a marathon."

O: Skin: moderately pale and cyanotic; respiratory distress no longer present; no spontaneous, uncontrolled cough noted; strong, nonproductive cough on request; vital signs: BP 135/85, HR 80, RR 10, T 37° C (98.6° F); palpation and percussion: negative; normal vesicular breath sounds in lower lung fields; ABGs (on 1 L/min O_2 by nasal cannula): pH 7.42, $Paco_2$ 72, HCO_3^- 45, Pao_2 78; Spo_2 94%

A: • Tuberculosis; (positive tuberculin reaction and acid-fast sputum stains)
• Chronic ventilatory failure with mild or corrected hypoxemia: normal for this patient (current ABGs, compared with outpatient baseline 6 months earlier)

P: Discontinue Oxygen Therapy, Bronchial Hygiene Therapy, and Hyperinflation Therapy Protocols. Discuss with patient need for chest clinic follow-up in 2 weeks and smoking-cessation program. Confirm follow-up arrangements with public health nurse who will visit patient at the Samaritan Shelter. Recheck ABGs on room air in chest clinic in 2 weeks.

DISCUSSION

Recent years have seen a disconcerting rise in the number of active cases of tuberculosis, particularly among the poor, the homeless, those living in crowded urban settings, and those with various degrees of immune suppression. A homeless, alcoholic patient with cough, fever, and hemoptysis is, of course, highly suggestive of tuberculosis.

A chest x-ray that shows a pneumonic infiltrate with cavity formation nearly makes the diagnosis, long before the results of the sputum acid-fast smear and tuberculin skin test are in hand. Most clinical cases of tuberculosis are not associated with gas exchange difficulties; however, that this patient presented with cyanosis, hypoxemia, a degree of carbon dioxide retention, and more than a few pulmonary infiltrates suggests that pulmonary tuberculosis may be only *one* of his respiratory diagnoses.

The patient's fever and tachypnea reflect his stimulated immune response and oxygen receptors stimulated by significant hypoxia. Auscultated rhonchi reflect **excessive bronchial secretions,** and bronchial breath sounds reflect lung **consolidation** and **atelectasis** (see Figs. 1-12, 1-9, and 1-8). The restrictive pathophysiology found in his pulmonary function tests (PFTs) reflects his decreased lung compliance caused by the pneumonic consolidation and atelectasis. That the patient demonstrates acute alveolar hyperventilation superimposed on chronic ventilatory failure verifies the advanced stage of the disorder and that impending ventilatory failure is certainly a possibility and concern.

Note that in the **first assessment** the patient has significant carboxyhemoglobinemia; thus his saturation when corrected for his carbon monoxide level is considerably lower than the pulse oximetry-determined hemoglobin saturation of 88% (in truth, $88 - 8.5 = 79.5\%$). Also note in the first assessment that the therapist picks up on the patient's secretions and history of smoking and places him on a vigorous program of bronchial hygiene therapy, which could consist of metered dose inhaler (MDI)–administered bronchodilators and mucolytics if indicated. Moreover, treatment should be aggressive at first because the patient complains of respiratory distress. Due to the finding of a cavity in an undiagnosed patient, careful chest physical therapy with percussion and postural drainage to that area of the lung is indicated. The patient's hypoxemia probably could be treated with low-flow oxygen therapy with careful monitoring of subsequent blood gases to ensure that carbon dioxide retention does not develop.

In addition, note that in the handling of the first part of this case the patient is not isolated properly, given the history and x-ray findings. Another caveat is that the bronchoscopic secretions are examined appropriately for malignant cells, as well as for routine and acid-fast organisms (the first because of the patient's cigarette smoking history and the second because of the by-then-recognized probability that the staff is dealing with active tuberculosis).

A final caveat is that if possible the patient should enter a good rehabilitation program where smoking cessation and nutrition counseling are readily available. Because his blood gases are so borderline, rechecking them during his time as an outpatient on low-flow oxygen certainly is indicated.

Chapter 10   *Fungal Diseases of the Lungs*

Response 1

S: "I feel short of breath, and my joints are swollen and painful."

O: Cyanosis; cough: frequent and strong, producing moderate amounts of thick, yellow sputum; vital signs: BP 160/90, HR 93, RR 18, T 37.8° C (100° F); palpation: red lesions on anterior chest and left cheek; auscultation: bilateral crackles and rhonchi in lung apices; CXR: bilateral fibrosis and calcification and spherical nodules; two to three 1- to 3-cm cavities in both upper lobes; ABGs (room air): pH 7.51, $PaCO_2$ 29, HCO_3^- 22, PaO_2 64

A: • Moderate respiratory distress (cyanosis, vital signs)
 • Excesive amounts of thick, yellow bronchial secretions (sputum, rhonchi)
    Infection likely (yellow sputum)
 • Pulmonary fibrosis, calcification, and cavities (CXR)
 • Acute alveolar hyperventilation with mild hypoxemia (ABGs)

P: Initiate Oxygen Therapy Protocol (e.g., 2 lpm per nasal cannula) and Bronchial Hygiene Therapy Protocol (e.g., C&DB instruction, PD to both upper lobes q-shift ×3 days). Order sputum culture (routine, AFB, and fungal). Encourage fluid intake. Monitor (e.g., oximeter, I&O).

Response 2

S: "I still can't get a good breath of air."

O: Respiratory distress: cyanotic, short of breath; positive spherulin skin test; coccidioidomycosis organisms seen in sputum smear; frequent strong cough: moderate amount of thick, opaque sputum; vital signs: BP 165/95, HR 97, RR 24, T normal; bilateral crackles and rhonchi in the lung apices; SpO_2 88%; ABGs: pH 7.54, $PaCO_2$ 27, HCO_3^- 21, PaO_2 55.

A: • Coccidioidomycosis (positive spherulin skin test, sputum smear)
 • Continued respiratory distress (cyanosis, vital signs)
 • Excessive amounts of thick bronchial secretions (sputum, rhonchi)
 • Acute alveolar hyperventilation with moderate hypoxemia (worsening ABGs)

P: Increase Oxygen Therapy Protocol (e.g., 3 lpm nasal cannula). Add Aerosolized Medication Protocol; up-regulate Bronchial Hygiene Therapy Protocol (e.g., 2 cc 10% acetylcysteine with 0.2 cc albuterol q6h followed by C&DB and PD to both upper lobes). Add supervised use of flutter valve 2×/shift. Request repeat CXR. Continue to monitor and reevaluate.

Response 3

S: "I'm breathing much better."

O: No obvious respiratory distress; no spontaneous cough; strong, nonproductive cough on request; vital signs: BP 135/88, HR 80, RR 14, T normal; bilateral crackles in the lung apices; SpO_2 91%; ABGs: pH 7.44, $PaCO_2$ 34, HCO_3^- 23, PaO_2 71

A: • Adequate bronchial hygiene status (nonproductive cough, absence of rhonchi, crackles expected in lung fibrosis)
  • Normal acid-base status with mild hypoxemia (ABGs)

P: Discontinue Oxygen Therapy Protocol. Recheck SpO_2 on room air ("spot check") in 1 hour. Discontinue Bronchial Hygiene Therapy Protocol. Instruct patient in trial use of Combivent (albuterol/ipratropium) MDI. Reevaluate off all therapy modalities but on self-administered MDI in AM; then sign off.

DISCUSSION

Respiratory care practitioners (RCPs) who work in the Southwest, where coccidioidomycosis is endemic, would probably anticipate the diagnosis in the patient with bilateral pulmonary infiltrates, swollen tender joints, and the typical skin rash of this lesion. Others could not be blamed if they missed this fact until the coccidioidal skin test came back positive and the sputum fungal smear demonstrated the coccidioidomycosis organism. In this case the patient demonstrated the clinical manifestations associated with the following two anatomic alterations of the lungs: **increased alveolar-capillary membrane thickness** (e.g., bilateral fibrosis and calcification; see Fig. 1-10) and **excessive bronchial secretions** (e.g., cough, sputum, and rhonchi; see Fig. 1-12).

The **first assessment**—that the patient is hypoxemic despite alveolar hyperventilation and that he has alveolar fibrosis and cavity formation—is correct. For the hypoxemia, oxygen therapy is appropriate and should be started with a nasal oxygen cannula at 1 to 2 L/min and then regulated with a pulse oximeter. In treating this case, as with any other pneumonia, the assessing RCP should quickly obtain a sputum, Gram stain, and acid-fast bacillus and fungal preparations; this step was appropriately done in this case. The treating RCP would do well to understand the use of tuberculin and fungal testing in such patients and to understand, as with other pneumonic infiltrates, that the therapist's impact once that is done would probably be minimal.

In the **second assessment** 4 days later the offending organism has been isolated and appropriate therapy with intravenous amphotericin-B started. The patient is still hypoxemic, and up-regulation of his oxygen therapy (perhaps to 3 or 4 L/min, or with a nonrebreathing mask if the former is unsuccessful) is indicated. Because the patient is still coughing up thick, opaque sputum and because his dyspnea is not relieved so far, up-regulation of the bronchial hygiene therapy program with a trial of bronchodilator therapy and mucolytic therapy is in order. Because the patient is not improving, a repeat chest x-ray appears indicated.

At the **last assessment** 10 days after the patient's admission to the hospital, clear improvement is noted. Oximetry reveals good peripheral oxygen saturation, and the blood gases are much improved. Now is the time for the treating therapist to reduce the intensity of the patient's respiratory care, and this step is illustrated in the appropriate response for this section of the case study. Follow-up pulmonary function testing 6 to 12 months after the abatement of acute illness would be worthwhile.

Chapter 11   Pulmonary Edema

Response 1

S: "I don't think I'm having a serious problem."

O: Vital signs: BP 100/50, HR 145 and irregular, RR 22, T normal; SpO_2 70%; anxiety and cough: small amount of frothy, pink secretions; bilateral, dull percussion notes over the lower lung areas; bilateral inspiratory crackles and expiratory wheezes over the lower lobes; ABGs (2 L/min O_2 by nasal cannula): pH 7.56, $Paco_2$ 28, HCO_3^- 20, Pao_2 51; CXR: dense, fluffy opacities in lower lungs; left cardiac enlargement

A: • Respiratory distress (vital signs, ABGs)
   • Hypotension (blood pressure)
   • Acute pulmonary edema (crackles, distended neck veins, CXR)
   • Acute alveolar hyperventilation with moderate hypoxemia (ABGs)
   • Small airway secretions, alveolar flooding, interstitial edema or any combination of these (crackles)
   • Bronchospasm?? (wheezing most likely caused by airway secretions)

P: Initiate Oxygen Therapy Protocol (e.g., increasing oxygenation to 50% Venturi mask). Hyperinflation Therapy Protocol (e.g., 5 cm H_2O CPAP mask qid for 15-30 min, or Bipap therapy at IPAP = 6 cm H_2O, EPAP = 4 cm H_2O; or if not tolerated, IPPB treatments for 15-30 min ×3). Begin Bronchial Hygiene Therapy Protocol (e.g., suctioning orally prn). Begin trial period of Aerosolized Medication Protocol (albuterol 0.25 cc in 2 cc normal saline qid). Monitor (e.g., vital signs, pulse oximetry, ABGs, cardiac enzymes and troponin levels) and reevaluate.

Response 2

S: "I still don't feel great."

O: Vital signs: BP 160/90, HR 105 and regular, RR 20, T 37.1° C (98.8° F); slight improvement in cyanosis; distended neck veins persistent; urine output: 650 ml last 2 hours; frequent, nonproductive cough; bilateral inspiratory crackles and expiratory wheezes over lower lobes; SpO_2 84%; ABGs: pH 7.54, $Paco_2$ 25, HCO_3^- 18, Pao_2 51

A: • Continued respiratory distress (vital signs, ABGs)
   • Improved systemic hypotension (BP)
   • Persistent acute pulmonary edema (physical findings, CXR)
   • Worsening acute alveolar hyperventilation with moderate hypoxemia—more severe than admission (ABGs)
   • Small airway secretions (crackles)
   • Bronchospasm?? (wheezing most likely caused by airway secretions)

P: Up-regulate Oxygen Therapy Protocol (e.g., increasing Fio_2 to 0.60). Up-regulate Hyperinflation Therapy Protocol (e.g., 10 cm H_2O CPAP mask qid for 15-30 min, or continuation of IPPB for 15 min). Continue Bronchial Hygiene Therapy Protocol (e.g., suction orally prn). Continue trial period of Aerosolized Medication Protocol as earlier. Continue to monitor closely (e.g., vital signs, pulse oximetry, ABGs).

Response 3

S: "I'm breathing better."

O: Vital signs: BP 140/115, HR 95 and regular, RR 16, T 37.3° C (99.1° F); no cyanosis; urine output: 850 ml over past 2 hours; neck veins no longer distended; cough: strong, nonproductive; bilateral crackles over lower lobes; SpO_2 97%; ABGs: pH 7.44, $PaCO_2$ 36, HCO_3^- 24, PaO_2 190

A: • Pulmonary edema (history and physical findings)
　　Condition appearing to improve
　• Small airway secretions (crackles)
　• Normal ventilatory/acid-base status with overly corrected hypoxemia (ABGs)

P: Down-regulate Oxygen Therapy Protocol (e.g., 2 lpm per nasal cannula). Discontinue Hyperinflation Therapy Protocol (however, continuation of incentive spirometry tid still appropriate). Discontinue Bronchial Hygiene Therapy and Aerosolized Medication Protocols. Continue to monitor and evaluate (e.g., vital signs, SpO_2 ABGs in AM).

DISCUSSION

The patient's known cardiac history, cough productive of foamy, pink-tinged sputum, neck vein distension, peripheral edema, and rapid atrial fibrillation are virtually pathognomonic of acute pulmonary edema. The therapist should be aware that the following conditions may precipitate pulmonary edema in a given patient:

1. Acute myocardial infarction
2. Hypertension
3. Valvular heart disease
4. Rapid ventricular rate with inadequate filling time of atria and ventricles
5. Exogenous fluid overload

In this case the patient demonstrated clinical manifestations associated with the following two specific anatomic alterations of the lungs: **increased alveolar-capillary membrane thickness** (e.g., dense, fluffy opacities in lower lungs and low PaO_2; see Fig. 1-10 and to a milder extent **excessive bronchial secretions** (e.g., frothy, pink secretions and crackles see Fig. 1-12).

The treatment of this condition involves oxygen therapy, maintenance of alveolar volume with positive end-expiratory pressure (PEEP) or continuous positive airway pressure (CPAP) therapy, and bronchial hygiene therapy directed at mechanical removal of secretions from the airway. In the past ethanol has been added to the inspirate to "reduce surface tension of the bubbles in the secretions," but this technique is falling from favor. Although trial periods may be appropriate, bronchodilator therapy typically is not required because smooth muscle bronchospasm usually does not occur in this condition.

In the **first assessment** the therapist may well have mentioned an interest in cardiac enzymes because treatment of the patient with acute myocardial infarction causing pulmonary edema is somewhat different than that of the other conditions mentioned previously.

After the **second assessment** the patient is clearly not doing well, his Pa_{O_2} is still low, and now the question of a coincident metabolic acidosis arises. This question is not uncommon in patients with cardiac disease who may be hypotensive. The blood gas observed in this case is more worrisome because the Pa_{O_2} is low despite alveolar hyperventilation. If the patient were not tolerating mask CPAP, intubation for intervention of PEEP therapy would be indicated at this point. If the patient were not already in the intensive care unit (ICU), transfer there at this point would be indicated.

After the **third assessment** this case highlights the rapid therapeutic response that can occur in most patients with pulmonary edema. Even patients with acute myocardial infarction as the cause of their pulmonary edema generally improve rapidly with therapy, such as outlined in this case. The cardiac inotropic and chronotropic agents and the intravenous diuretic therapy started in the emergency room 9 hours or so earlier have by this time exerted their maximal effect. If monitoring of pulse oximetry and blood gases in the next 24 hours continues to provide reassuring results, the therapist can probably sign off this case and the patient can go on his planned trip to Alaska.

KEY POINT ANSWERS

For Pulmonary Edema (DRG* 127)

1. Basic Concept Formation
   a. *Yes.* When the pump action of the left heart fails, pulmonary venous drainage is impaired and first interstitial and then alveolar edema occur. The body perceives this failure through several mechanisms (see answer 2.b) and responds with a sensation of dyspnea.
   b. The pulmonary venous pressure *increases* when the pump action of the left heart fails.
   c. The word *edema* comes from the Greek *oidema,* meaning *swelling.*
   d. *Smoking, obesity,* and *age* are common risk factors for both heart and lung disease.
2. Database Formation
   a. In cases of mild or early pulmonary edema, *alveolar-capillary membrane swelling* and thickening with edema fluid occur. In more advanced cases, *alveolar flooding* with edema fluid occurs.† This fluid may fill the airways up to the oropharynx, where it is clinically called *foaming pulmonary edema.* The reader may note similarities between this pathologic process and that of near drowning.‡
   b. Increased alveolar-capillary membrane thickness results in alveolar diffusion blockade. The lung is stiff and waterlogged and demonstrates reduced compliance (see Fig. 1-10). Relative shunt physiology develops as alveolar flooding occurs. Hypoxemia drives various oxygen and pressure receptors, which increase both heart rate and ventilatory rate. If the cardiac output is *not limited* by intrinsic heart disease, cardiac output may increase.
   c. (See answer 2.b). Vascular markings would increase, progressing to *"white out" of the chest x-ray* as the pulmonary edema worsens. *Bronchial breath sounds* and *crackles* would be heard. *Restrictive pathologic* processes would be observed on pulmonary function testing. *Hypoxemia* despite alveolar hyperventilation would be noted.
   d. *Chest pain, orthopnea, paroxysmal nocturnal dyspnea,* and *peripheral edema* are common signs and symptoms of congestive heart failure and pulmonary edema. *Systemic hypertension* may be noted and indeed is a common cause of left ventricular failure. Various left-sided *cardiac murmurs* may reflect aortic or mitral valvular disease as the cause of the patient's pulmonary edema. *Gallop cardiac rhythms* may suggest *cardiomyopathy* as the cause of the heart failure. Signs of *hypothyroidism* may provide clues to myxedematous cardiomyopathy.
   e. The main goals of therapy are *reduction of pulmonary venous* and *left ventricular end-diastolic pressure, relief of dyspnea,* and *treatment of hypoxemia.* If *ventilatory failure* occurs, *support of alveolar ventilation* is an additional goal.
   f. Following are standard therapist-driven protocols (TDPs) that might achieve these goals:
      1. Pharmacologic means are available to reduce pulmonary venous hypertension and left ventricular end-diastolic pressure. These means are *not* in the standard respiratory care practitioner's armamentarium. They include antihypertensives, antiarrhythmic agents, diuretics, and cardiac inotropic and

---

DRG, Diagnosis-related group.
†*See color plate 12 in Des Jardins T, Burton GG: Clinical manifestations and assessment of respiratory disease, ed 4, St. Louis, 2002, Mosby.*
‡*See color plate 35 in Des Jardins T, Burton GG: Clinical manifestations and assessment of respiratory disease, ed 4, St. Louis, 2002, Mosby.*

KEY POINT ANSWERS—cont'd

chronotropic agents. Their effects are evaluated in the acutely ill by *pulmonary artery* (Swan-Ganz) *catheter monitoring,* a task which is in the job description of many critical care, institutionally certified respiratory-care practitioners (RCPs).

2. The treatment of dyspnea in these patients is often difficult. The *Oxygen Therapy Protocol* (see Protocol 1-1) is absolutely necessary and may sometimes only be effective when used with continuous positive airway pressure *(CPAP)* in the *Hyperinflation Therapy Protocol* (see Protocol 1-3).

3. If ventilatory failure develops, mechanical ventilation therapy is used in conjunction with positive end-expiratory pressure (PEEP) therapy in the Hyperinflation Therapy Protocol (see Protocol 1-3).

g. Following are the outcomes, adverse effects, and monitors of the preceding protocols:

1. The *outcomes* desired include improvement in hypoxemia to SaO_2 less than 92% and treatment of acute ventilatory failure with early extubation if ventilatory management become necessary.

2. The only *adverse effect* worth noting in this selection of therapies is *barotrauma* secondary to high mean airway pressures.

3. Appropriate *monitors* in acute pulmonary edema include the following:
   a. SpO_2
   b. ECG rate, rhythm, and morphology
   c. Pulmonary capillary wedge pressure
   d. Intake and output records and daily weights
   e. Serial chest x-ray films
   f. Careful monitoring of mean airway pressure in ventilated patients
   g. Weaning parameters if extubation is contemplated

3. Assessment

   a. *Yes.* He had a history of *hypertension, cigarette smoking,* and *atrial fibrillation* recently.

   b. *Yes.* He had tachycardia, atrial fibrillation with a rapid ventricular response, tachypnea, cyanosis, foamy, pink tracheal secretions, and severe peripheral edema. Auscultation of the chest revealed crackles. His chest x-ray showed cardiomegaly and the centrally dense hilar infiltrates typical of the disorder.

   c. *Yes.* His dyspnea reflected his *alveolar-capillary block and decreased lung compliance.*

   d. Literally *all* the manifestations listed previously indicate that he was severely, if not critically, ill.

4. Application

   a. Oxygen therapy *was* indicated because of his *cardiac irritability* and significant *hypoxemia* despite alveolar hyperventilation. Morphine sulfate is often given for treatment of acute pulmonary edema. If the patient's hyperventilation stopped as a result of such therapy, his PaO_2 would drop further.

   b. *Monitoring was* indicated for *all* the reasons listed in answer 2.g.

   c. The use of *bronchial hygiene therapy* in this case *is open to debate.* He did have a "small" amount of secretions and wheezes on admission, and certainly *deep breathing and coughing* and *suctioning* as required would be appropriate then.

   d. Because of their cardiac irritability potential, *bronchodilators* must be used with caution in patients with cardiac disease. There were no clear indications.

e. *Hyperinflation therapy was* indicated to increase and stabilize alveolar size.
f. Mechanical ventilation *was not* indicated in this patient because he tolerated the CPAP begun at the time of the *second assessment,* and CO_2 retention never developed.

5. Evaluation
   a. Skillful oxygen and hyperinflation therapy should *improve hypoxemia and decrease the alveolar-arterial oxygen gradient.* The *heart rate and respiratory rate should fall.*
   b. Look for *improvement in all monitors* discussed in answer 2.g. Improvement in the chest x-ray may lag behind improvement in static compliance and arterial blood gases (ABGs).
   c. *Mask oxygen therapy* can be increased to an FIO_2 of 1.0. *Mask CPAP* tolerances vary, but 12 to 15 cm H_2O is at the upper limit of most individuals' tolerance. *PEEP pressures* in excess of 15 cm H_2O are associated with an increased risk of *barotrauma.*
   d. *Mask or cannula oxygen therapy* is inexpensive and relatively safe (remote risk in this case of oxygen toxicity or hypoventilation). *Mask CPAP* is not well tolerated by most individuals but is certainly less invasive and less costly then intubation and *mechanical ventilation.* A *pulmonary artery catheter* carries the risk of infection, pneumothorax, arrhythmias, and embolization.
   e. Therapy in *ventilated* patients with pulmonary edema may be reduced (weaned) in the following order:
      1. Reduce PEEP pressures to 5 cm H_2O.
      2. Wean from pressure support.
      3. Extubate and put on mask FIO_2 5% to 10% higher than ventilator FIO_2.
      4. Titrate FIO_2.

6. Boundary Awareness
   a. His A-a oxygen gradient would worsen, and his PaO_2 *would fall.* His respiratory rate would *increase,* as would his *dyspnea.* His *weight would increase,* and he would be in *positive fluid balance.* His *chest x-ray* film would show increasing opacity.
   b. If any of the items in answer 6.a happen, ask a supervisor for help.
   c. Call the patient's physician before *intubation* of the patient.
   d. The $PaCO_2$ would rise, and *acute respiratory* (and possibly metabolic) *acidemia* would occur.
   e. See answer 5.d.

Chapter 12   *Pulmonary Embolism*

Response 1

S: "My breathing is OK."

O: No remarkable respiratory distress noted; vital signs: BP 115/75, HR 75, RR 11; afebrile; tenderness over left shoulder and left anterior chest area; normal vesicular breath sounds; CXR: normal; ABGs (partial rebreathing mask): pH 7.40, $Paco_2$ 41, HCO_3^- 24, Pao_2 504 mm Hg; Spo_2 97%

A: • No remarkable respiratory problems
   • Normal acid-base status with over-oxygenation

P: Reduce oxygen therapy per protocol (e.g., 2 lpm by nasal cannula). Recheck Spo_2 on room air.

Response 2

S: "I feel awful. I'm short of breath and lightheaded."

O: Cyanosis; agitation, and dyspnea; cough productive of small amount of blood-tinged sputum; vital signs: BP 90/45, HR 125, RR 30, T 37.2° C (99° F), slight wheezing throughout both lung fields; pleural friction rub, right middle lobe; ECG: normal sinus rhythm, sinus tachycardia, atrial flutter; hemodynamic indices: increased CVP, RAP, $\overline{PA}$, RVSWI, and PVR and decreased PCWP, CO, SV, SVI, and CI; CXR: atelectasis and consolidation in the right middle lobe; ABGs: pH 7.53, $Paco_2$ 26, HCO_3^- 21 mmol/L, Pao_2 53 mm Hg; Spo_2 89%

A: • Hypotension (BP)
   • Respiratory distress (cyanosis, heart rate, respiratory rate, ABGs)
   • Pulmonary embolism and infarction likely (history, vital signs, CXR, ECG, blood-tinged sputum, wheezing, pleural friction rub)
   • Bronchospasm, probably secondary to pulmonary embolism or infarction (wheezing)
   • Alveolar atelectasis and consolidation (CXR)
   • Acute alveolar hyperventilation with moderate hypoxemia (ABGs)
   • Pulmonary artery hypertension and low cardiac output probably secondary to pulmonary embolism (clinical presentation and hemodynamic data)

P: Contact physician to request transfer to ICU. Increase oxygen therapy per protocol (e.g., 4 lpm by nasal cannula). Begin Aerosolized Medication Protocol (e.g., med. neb. with 2 cc albuterol premix qid). Monitor and reevaluate in 30 minutes (e.g., ABG). Remain on standby with mechanical ventilator.

Response 3

S: N/A (patient not responsive)

O: Ventilation-perfusion scan: no blood flow to right middle lobe; cyanosis; cough: small amount of blood-tinged sputum; vital signs: BP 70/35, HR 160, RR 25 and shallow, T 37.5° C (99.2° F); palpation negative; dull percussion notes over right middle lobe; wheezing over both lung fields; pleural friction rub over right middle lobe; ECG: alternating among normal sinus rhythm, sinus tachycardia, and atrial flutter; hemodynamic indices: increased CVP, RAP, PA, RVSWI, and PVR and decreased PCWP, CO, SV, SVI, and CI; ABGs: pH 7.25, $PaCO_2$ 69, HCO_3^- 27, PaO_2 37; SpO_2 64%

A: • Pulmonary embolism and infarction (history, vital signs, hemodynamics, CXR, ECG, blood-tinged sputum, wheezing, pleural friction rub)
• Continued respiratory distress (heart rate, respiratory rate, ABGs)
• Bronchospasm (wheezing)
• Acute ventilatory failure with severe hypoxemia (ABGs)

P: Contact physician stat. Discuss acute ventilatory failure and need for intubation and mechanical ventilation. Increase Oxygen Therapy Protocol (e.g., increasing O_2 to 100% pending physician's orders). Increase Aerosolized Medication Protocol (e.g., changing med. nebs. to IPPB to assist patient's work of breathing q4h).

DISCUSSION

Risk factors for development of a fatal pulmonary embolism include immobilization, malignant disease, and a history of thrombotic disease (including venous thrombosis) congestive heart failure, and chronic lung disease. Only about 10% of patients with pulmonary emboli do *not* have at least one of these risk factors. The symptoms of ultimately fatal pulmonary embolism include dyspnea (in about 60% of patients), syncope (in about 25%), altered mental status, apprehension, nonpleuritic chest pain, sweating, cough, and hemoptysis (in a smaller percentage of patients).

The signs of acute pulmonary embolism include tachypnea, tachycardia, crackles, low-grade temperature, lower extremity edema, hypotension, cyanosis, gallop rhythm, diaphoresis, and clinically evident phlebitis (in a small percentage of patients).

The diagnosis of thromboembolic disease is most often made with ventilation-perfusion lung scanning, although pulmonary angiography remains the "gold standard" for diagnosis. Impedance plethysmography or duplex ultrasonography or venography of the extremities is helpful when embolic disease is suspected from venous thrombosis in the extremities.

Interesting to note is that in surgical patients at least half the deaths due to pulmonary embolism occur within the first week after the surgical procedure, most commonly on the third to seventh day after the operation. The remainder of the deaths, however, divide equally among the second, third, and fourth postoperative weeks. The current patient certainly has one of the obvious causes for pulmonary embolism, namely immobilization of the left leg, which was put in a cast after surgery.

At the time of the **first assessment** the patient is not in any respiratory distress. His chest physical examination is basically unremarkable, as are the chest x-ray and arterial blood gases. The patient might well have been placed on hyperexpansion therapy, as with incentive spirometry, because his known fractures were expected to be surgically reduced. This fact is particularly important in this patient, who was on morphine and may be tempted to hypoventilate because of his left shoulder and left anterior chest pain and tenderness.

By the time of the **second assessment,** however, things have changed, and the patient demonstrates many of the signs and symptoms listed previously. The assessing therapist should recognize the seriousness of the situation from the patient's complaints, physical findings, hemodynamic parameters, and arterial blood gases. The patient's wheezing is most likely due to pulmonary embolism and infarction, as is the alveolar atelectasis. However, a trial of aerosolized bronchodilation is not inappropriate. The data are abnormal enough to prompt the therapist to suggest that the patient be transferred to the intensive care unit and to prepare for ventilator standby because acute ventilatory failure may not be far off.

Indeed in the **last assessment,** things have progressed to the point at which the patient is in severe respiratory acidemia with severe hypoxemia, and mechanical ventilation becomes necessary. The treating therapist should recognize that the therapeutic options in these cases are limited by the amount of ventilation "wasted" in such patients because of their embolic disease. High-minute ventilation may be necessary to improve (even slightly) the arterial blood gases in such patients.

A final note is that wheezing due to pulmonary embolic disease is relatively rare, occurring in less than 2% of hospitalized patients. The outlook for this patient is extremely poor. Indeed in the fifth week of this hospitalization the patient died. He remained on ventilatory support until the time of his death.

Chapter 13   *Flail Chest*

Response 1

S: N/A (patient unconscious)

O: Vital signs: BP 165/92, HR 120, RR 26 and shallow, T 36.2° C (97.2° F); paradoxical movement of the anterior chest wall; skin: pale and cyanotic; diminished breath sounds bilaterally; CXR: multiple double rib fractures of the right and left anterior and lateral ribs, between ribs 4 and 9; sternum fractured in three places; atelectasis bilaterally; ABGs (nonrebreathing mask): pH 7.17, $PaCO_2$ 82, HCO_3^- 27, PaO_2 37; SpO_2 59%

A: • Flail chest (paradoxical chest movement, CXR)
• Atelectasis bilaterally (CXR)
• Acute ventilatory failure with severe hypoxemia (ABGs)
• Acute alcohol intoxication with near-fatal blood alcohol level

P: Initiate mechanical ventilation per protocol–stat. Also begin hyperinflation and oxygenation therapies per protocols. Monitor and reevaluate (e.g., in 1 hour).

Response 2

S: N/A

O: Cyanotic and pale appearance; distended neck veins; vital signs: BP 100/65, HR 145, RR 12 (controlled), T unchanged; auscultation: right lung, absent breath sounds and left lung, diminished breath sounds, rhonchi, and crackles; CXR: left lung, partially aerated and patches of atelectasis; right lung, completely atelectatic; hemodynamic indices: increased CVP, RAP, $\overline{PA}$, RVSWI, and PVR and decreased PCWP, $\dot{C}O$, SV, SVI, CI, LVSWI, and SVR; oxygenation indices: increased $\dot{Q}s/\dot{Q}T$, $C(a - \overline{v})O_2$, and O_2ER and decreased DO_2 and SvO_2; ABGs: pH 7.25, $PaCO_2$ 65, HCO_3^- 25, PaO_2 54; SpO_2 86%

A: • Atelectasis: patches throughout left lung; right lung airless (CXR)
• Increased pulmonary vascular resistance and decreased cardiac output (distended neck veins, hemodynamic indices)
• Acute ventilatory failure with moderate hypoxemia (ABGs)
• Poor oxygenation status (oxygenation indices)

P: Contact physician regarding patient's hemodynamic and oxygenation status; consider therapeutic bronchoscopy to treat atelectasis. Up-regulate mechanical ventilation per protocol to decrease $PaCO_2$ (e.g., increasing rate or volume). Up-regulate hyperinflation therapy per protocol (e.g., increasing PEEP). Up-regulate oxygenation therapy per protocol (if not already at an FIO_2 of 1). Monitor and reevaluate (e.g., in 30 to 60 minutes).

Response 3

S: N/A

O: Cyanotic skin and distended neck veins; vital signs: BP 80/32, HR 190, RR 14 (controlled), T 38.9° C (102° F); right lung: no breath sounds; left lung: rhonchi and crackles; large amounts of yellow sputum; ECG: premature ventricular contractions; CXR: left lung partially aerated with patches of atelectasis (worsening) and right lung airless; early signs of ARDS; hemodynamics: worsening; ABGs: pH 7.22, $PaCO_2$ 71, HCO_3^- 24, PaO_2 34; oxygenation status: worsening; SpO_2 61%

A: • Atelectasis: patches throughout left lung (worsening); right lung completely atelectatic (CXR)
  • Early stages of ARDS (CXR)
  • Excessive bronchial secretions (sputum, rhonchi)
    Infection likely (yellow sputum)
  • Increased pulmonary vascular resistance and decreased cardiac output: worsening (distended neck veins, hemodynamic indices)
  • Acute ventilatory failure with severe hypoxemia (ABGs)
  • Poor oxygenation status: worsening (oxygenation indices)

P: Contact physician regarding patient's hemodynamic and oxygenation status; consider bronchoscopy. Up-regulate mechanical ventilation (if possible) per protocol to decrease $PaCO_2$ (e.g., increasing in rate or volume). Up-regulate hyperinflation therapy per protocol. Discuss with physician possible use of super-PEEP with pressures >20 cm H_2O. Up-regulate Oxygen Therapy Protocol, Bronchial Hygiene Therapy Protocol (e.g., albuterol premix 2 cc q4h), Aerosolized Medication Protocol (e.g., in-line 2 cc 20% acetylcysteine with 0.5 cc albuterol). Obtain sputum culture. Monitor and reevaluate frequently.

DISCUSSION

This patient demonstrates the sequelae of an abnormal chest wall or respiratory muscular pump. The uneven ventilation that resulted from his multiple chest fractures gave him an unstable (flail) chest, causing atelectasis to develop. Several clinical manifestations associated with **atelectasis** (see Fig. 1-8) were soon presented in this case. For example, the patient's decreased lung compliance was manifested in his tachycardia and tachypnea, whereas his hypoxemia reflected the efforts seen with classic **pulmonary shunting** (see Fig. 1-8). His condition was extremely severe, as demonstrated by his first arterial blood gas values—pH 7.17, $PaCO_2$ 82, HCO_3^- 27, and PaO_2 37.

In the **first assessment** the treating therapist correctly recognizes the patient's acute ventilatory failure, intubates him, and places him on mechanical ventilation per protocol. The patient's hypoxemia is treated by an increase in the inspired oxygen concentration, and an attempt should be made to stabilize the chest still further and treat his early **atelectasis** with positive end-expiratory pressure (PEEP) (see Fig. 1-8). Many cases treated in this manner achieve "stability" of the chest wall much sooner than one would expect, that is, within a few days. This case, however, is an exception.

The **second assessment** shows that the patient is developing signs of pulmonary hypertension with increased pulmonary vascular resistance and a low cardiac output. The right lung has become completely atelectatic despite ventilatory care. A recommendation for therapeutic bronchoscopy is certainly timely. More PEEP could be added to the ventilator settings, and higher tidal volumes might well be used in such a patient. His respiratory acidosis certainly must be treated more aggressively with a change in ventilator settings (e.g., by increasing the rate). Mechanical deadspace must be kept to a minimum in such patients.

The **third scenario** demonstrates that the patient has begun to slip into adult respiratory distress syndrome (ARDS) and that the atelectasis noted earlier is still a problem. His blood gases have worsened despite ventilator management, and the outlook has become increasingly grim. Repeat bronchoscopic examinations are often necessary in this situation, and a suggestion by the treating therapist that the procedure be repeated would be appropriate. If the sputum is thick, mucolytic agents may be added. Prompt culture of the sputum is an excellent idea because the organisms may have changed during the patient's hospital stay.

Despite the aggressive care this patient received, he died 24 hours later.

Chapter 14   Pneumothorax

Response 1

S: "I've been coughing so much and so hard my chest hurts."

O: Thin, but well nourished appearance; use of accessory muscles of respiration; cyanosis, digital clubbing, pursed-lip breathing, and barrel chest; cough: frequent, strong, and productive—large amounts of thick, yellow-green sputum; vital signs: BP 145/85, HR 94, RR 20, T 37.9° C (100.3° F); hyperresonant percussion notes bilaterally; diminished breath sounds and rhonchi bilaterally; expiration prolonged; diminished heart sounds; PFT (6 months previously): moderate-to-severe obstructive pulmonary disease; CXR: translucent, flattened hemidiaphragms and narrow heart; 10% pneumothorax between the second and third ribs on the left in the anterior axillary line; ABGs (room air): pH 7.53, $PaCO_2$ 48, HCO_3^- 38, PaO_2 57 (baseline: pH 7.42, $PaCO_2$ 69, HCO_3^- 41, PaO_2 74).

A: • Exacerbation of chronic bronchitis and emphysema (history, CXR)
• Respiratory distress (vital signs, ABGs)
• Left pneumothorax: 10% (CXR)
• Excessive bronchial secretions (sputum, rhonchi)
    Infection likely (yellow-green sputum)
• Acute alveolar hyperventilation superimposed on chronic ventilatory failure (ABGs, history)

P: Initiate Oxygen Therapy Protocol (e.g., HAFOE at FIO_2 of 0.28). Administer Aerosolized Medication Protocol (e.g., med. nebs. with 0.5 cc albuterol, in 2 cc 10% acetylcysteine, followed by bronchial hygiene therapy). Begin Bronchial Hygiene Therapy Protocol (e.g., PD while awake and sputum Gram's stain and culture). Monitor and reevaluate each shift.

Response 2

S: "I feel horrible."

O: Cyanosis, use of accessory muscles of respiration, and pursed-lip breathing; cough: frequent and weak; patient bracing himself when he coughs; small amount of yellow-green sputum; left anterior chest: hyperinflated and fixed; vital signs: BP 95/55, HR 125, RR 28 and shallow; hyperresonant notes bilaterally; right lung: diminished breath sounds and rhonchi; left lung: no breath sounds; diminished heart sounds over right lung field; CXR: large, left-sided pneumothorax with mediastinal shift rightward; ABGs: pH 7.24, $PaCO_2$ 103, HCO_3^- 43, PaO_2 37; SpO_2 62%

A: • Large, left-sided tension pneumothorax (CXR)
    Treatment with tube thoracotomy
• Respiratory distress (general appearance, vital signs, ABGs)
• Left lung: collapsed or atelectatic or both (CXR)
• Right lung: patches of atelectasis (CXR)
• Excessive bronchial secretions (sputum, rhonchi)
• Acute ventilatory failure superimposed on chronic ventilatory failure with severe hypoxemia (ABGs)

Response 2–cont'd

P: Contact physician to consider transfer to ICU. Continue Oxygen Therapy Protocol (e.g., FIO_2 at 0.8 and ABG checking in 30 minutes). Administer Bronchial Hygiene Therapy Protocol (e.g., continuing at present intensity; no physical therapy). Stay at patient's bedside. Do not perform mechanical ventilation per physician at present time (patient/physician directive). Perform Hyperinflation Therapy Protocol (e.g., low CPAP trial). Stay at patient's bedside. Monitor and reevaluate (e.g., in 30 minutes).

Response 3

S: "I'm feeling better."

O: CXR: left lung reexpansion about 75%; right lung: no patches of atelectasis; cyanosis no longer present; pursed-lip breathing and use of accessory muscles of respiration; right lung: rhonchi and diminished breath sounds; left lung: diminished breath sounds; vital signs: BP 145/85, HR 105, RR 22, T 38° C (100.5° F); hyperresonant notes bilaterally; ABGs: pH 7.35, $PaCO_2$ 85, HCO_3^- 41, PaO_2 64; SpO_2 90%

A: • Left-sided pneumothorax: improving (CXR)
  • 25% left lung collapse or atelectasis: improving (CXR)
  • Excessive bronchial secretions (rhonchi, earlier SOAPs)
  • Chronic ventilatory failure with severe hypoxemia (ABGs)
    ABGs not at patient's baseline level yet

P: Continue present level of Hyperinflation Therapy Protocol (e.g., CPAP mask). Continue present level of Oxygen Therapy Protocol. Continue present level of bronchial hygiene therapy per protocol. Monitor and reevaluate (e.g., in 4 to 6 hours).

DISCUSSION

The causes of pneumothorax include trauma to the chest wall, malignancy, infection of the pleural space or lung, rupture of subpleural bullas, and air leakage from tuberculous foci. The condition also may be without known cause (idiopathic). Pneumothoraces may be caused iatrogenically by needle tears of the pleura incurred during percutaneous needle lung biopsy or during aspiration of air or fluid from the pleural space.

This case demonstrates a pneumothorax caused by infection in a patient known to have chronic obstructive pulmonary disease (COPD). A rupture of a subpleural bulla or leakage of air from a parenchymal lung bulla may have accounted for his problem. The patient had pneumonia 4 years previously. If the pneumonia was due to a necrotizing organism, it could have weakened the visceral pleura, allowing air leakage. However, 4 years seems a bit long for that condition to be showing up at the current admission.

In the **first assessment** the therapist's attention to the patient's worsening pulmonary function is appropriate. Increasing his oxygenation by use of a Venturi oxygen mask would be acceptable, as would a trial of low-flow nasal cannula oxygen. The readers who recognized the small pneumothorax and noted it regarding specific boundaries for bronchial hygiene therapy are certainly worthy of praise. The readers who moved to obtain an early sputum culture, knowing that prompt treatment of infection would be helpful, also deserve commendation.

Despite this action, **3 hours later** the patient is clearly worsening, and indeed a stat has been called. The patient's chest x-ray film demonstrates a left tension pneumothorax, and the therapist at this point can ensure that a tube thoracostomy setup is available for the physician. Bilateral **atelectasis** is present, reflected in the crackles, chest radiograph, cyanosis, and low PaO_2 (see Fig. 1-8). The respiratory care practitioner's (RCP's) assessment would come after the chest tube has been placed and is functioning well, and he or she would so record that fact in the assessment. The RCP should note that the compressive atelectasis noted earlier has improved and help honor the patient's and physician's requests to avoid use of a ventilator if at all possible. However, the patient's CO_2 probably is high enough (103 mm Hg) to preclude this action. A trial of a respiratory stimulant, such as doxapram (Dopram), might be used in this setting. The therapist may try to increase the end-expiratory pressure to treat the atelectasis, but the reader should know that such therapy is fraught with the possibility of air-trapping in patients with obstructive pulmonary disease.

Chapter 15   Pleural Diseases

Response 1

S: "I cannot take a deep breath."

O: Malnourished appearance with poor personal hygiene; cyanosis with an occasional hacking, nonproductive cough; vital signs: BP 146/92, HR 112, RR 36 and shallow, T 37.7° C (99.8° F); trachea slightly shifted to the left; dull percussion notes over the right middle and right lower lobes; normal vesicular breath sounds over the left lung fields and right upper lobe; no breath sounds over the right middle and right lower lobes; CXR: large, right-sided pleural effusion, right middle and right lower lobes partially collapsed and consolidated; about 2 L of yellow fluid obtained via thoracentesis; ABGs (on 3 L/min O_2 by nasal cannula): pH 7.53, $Paco_2$ 24, HCO_3^- 19, Pao_2 37; Spo_2 44%

A: • Right-sided pneumonia and pleural effusion (CXR)
    Partially collapsed right middle and lower lobes; atelectasis versus pneumonia (CXR)
• Respiratory distress (vital signs, ABGs)
• Acute alveolar hyperventilation with severe hypoxemia (ABGs)
    Metabolic (lactic) acidosis likely (ABGs compared with Pco_2-HCO_3^--pH relationship nomogram)

P: Begin Hyperinflation Therapy Protocol (e.g., incentive spirometry q2h) and Oxygen Therapy Protocol (e.g., Fio_2 = 1.0 via nonrebreathing mask). Request nutrition consultation. Ensure thoracentesis fluid cultures are being obtained. Monitor and reevaluate.

Response 2

S: "I'm feeling better but not great yet."

O: Cyanotic and pale appearance; occasional dry, nonproductive cough; vital signs: BP 135/85, HR 100, RR 24, T normal; dull percussion notes over right middle and right lower lobes; normal vesicular breath sounds over left lung and over right upper lobe; bronchial breath sounds over right middle and lower lobes; CXR: small right-sided pleural effusion; right middle and right lower lobe consolidation; ABGs: pH 7.52, $Paco_2$ 29, HCO_3^- 22, Pao_2 57; Spo_2 89%

A: • Small right-sided pneumonia and pleural effusion, greatly improved (CXR)
    Atelectasis and consolidation in right middle and lower lung lobes (CXR)
• Continued respiratory distress, but improving (vital signs, ABGs)
• Acute alveolar hyperventilation with moderate hypoxemia, improved (ABGs)

P: Up-regulate hyperinflation therapy and oxygen therapy per respective protocols. Monitor and reevaluate.

Response 3

S: "I've finally caught my breath."

O: Relaxed, alert appearance, in semi-Fowler's position; paleness but no cyanosis; no spontaneous cough; vital signs: BP 128/79, HR 88, RR 16, T normal; dull percussion notes in right middle and right lower lung lobes; normal vesicular breath sounds over left lung and right upper lobe; bronchial breath sounds over right middle and right lower lobes; ABGs: pH 7.45, $Paco_2$ 36, HCO_3^- 24, Pao_2 77; Spo_2 92%

A: • Small, right-sided pneumonia and pleural effusion, greatly improved (previous CXR)
  Atelectasis and consolidation in right middle and right lower lung lobes (previous CXR)
• Normal acid-base status with mild hypoxemia (ABGs)

P: Maintain present levels of hyperinflation therapy and oxygen therapy per protocols. Monitor and reevaluate each shift.

DISCUSSION

This case illustrates a patient with pleural effusion, one of the pleural diseases that generally can be improved with appropriate therapy (in this case a 2-liter thoracentesis).

At the end of the **first assessment** the respiratory care practitioner recognizes that the patient has significant respiratory morbidity. Indeed the patient has extensive pneumonia and severe hypoxemia, despite alveolar hyperventilation. Understanding that **atelectasis** is the main pathophysiologic mechanism operating in this case (see Fig. 1-8), the practitioner correctly assesses the situation as one needing careful monitoring and begins oxygen therapy, presumably with a high concentration of oxygen in view of the patient's Pao_2. The practitioner recalls that the offending organism(s) is not yet identified and ensures that sputum and thoracentesis fluid cultures are obtained.

A trial of bronchial hygiene therapy would not be unwarranted in this case, given the patient's cigarette smoking history alone or the degree of severity of the condition. Admittedly, the physical findings in this patient (no wheeze or expiratory prolongation) did not indicate such therapy. Given the patient's history, the respiratory care practitioner also would be interested in the results of the cytologic studies for malignancy in both the sputum and thoracentesis fluid.

Frequently blood gases do not improve immediately after a thoracentesis, despite the fluid removal, because the atelectasis under the pleural effusion takes some time (hours or days) to dissipate. For this reason, hyperinflation therapy after thoracentesis is appropriate.

At the time of the **second assessment** the patient is beginning to improve, although she has signs of right middle and lower lobe consolidation. Good breath sounds are heard over the left lung and upper right lung, although bronchial breath sounds reflecting consolidation are still noted on the right. The respiratory therapist now should be concerned that atelectasis is still present and should increase the hyperinflation therapy with, perhaps, a positive expiratory pressure (PEP) mask or, possibly, with intensified incentive spirometry or intermittent positive-pressure breathing (IPPB).

In the **last assessment** the patient continues to do fairly well, although she is far from returning to baseline values. The persistent pneumonitis/atelectasis and mild hypoxemia, despite supplemental oxygen therapy, suggests the need for continued significant (though unchanged) therapy.

This case demonstrates that often in-place therapy *does not* need to be changed at each assessment. Indeed, this guide may apply to as many as 50% to 60% of accurately performed seriatim assessments. For pedagogic reasons, this option has not been exercised often in this text. However, this third assessment (in a patient with pleural effusion and underlying atelectasis/pneumonia) is a good case in point.

Chapter 16   Kyphoscoliosis

Response 1

S: "I'm having trouble breathing."

O: Well nourished appearance; severe anterior and left lateral curvature of the spine; cyanosis, digital clubbing, and distended neck veins—especially on the right side; cough: frequent, adequate, and productive of moderate amounts of thick yellow sputum; vital signs: BP 160/100, HR 90, RR 18, T 36.3° C (97.4° F); trachea deviated to the right; both lungs: dull percussion notes, crackles, and rhonchi; PFT: VC, FRC, and RV 45% to 50% of predicted; Hct 58%, Hb 18 g/dl; CXR: severe thoracic and spinous deformity, mediastinal shift, cardiomegaly, and bilateral infiltrates in the lung bases consistent with pneumonia or atelectasis; ABGs (room air): pH 7.52, $PaCO_2$ 58, HCO_3^- 42, PaO_2 49; SpO_2 78%

A: • Severe kyphoscoliosis (history, CXR, ABGs, physical examination)
  • Increased work of breathing (elevated blood pressure, heart rate, and respiratory rate)
  • Excessive bronchial secretions (sputum, rhonchi)
      Infection likely (thick, yellow sputum)
      Good ability to mobilize secretions (strong cough)
  • Atelectasis and consolidation (CXR)
  • Acute alveolar hyperventilation superimposed on chronic ventilatory failure with moderate hypoxemia (ABGs)
      Possible impending ventilatory failure
  • Cor pulmonale (CXR and physical examination)

P: Initiate Oxygen Therapy Protocol (HAFOE at FIO_2 0.28; care not to overoxygenate the patient) and Bronchial Hygiene Therapy Protocol (sputum for Gram's stain and culture; C&DB instructions and oral suction prn). Begin Hyperinflation Therapy Protocol (e.g., incentive spirometry qid and prn). Begin Aerosolized Medication Protocol (e.g., IPPB with aerosolized albuterol 0.5 cc in 1.5 cc 10% acetylcysteine q4h). Notify physician of admitting ABGs and possible ventilatory failure. Place mechanical ventilator on standby. When patient is stable, educate about possible future use of noninvasive positive pressure ventilation (NPPV). Monitor q1h × 8 hours, then 2×/shift if stable.

Response 2

S: Severe dyspnea; "I'm extremely short of breath."

O: Extreme respiratory distress; cyanosis and perspiration; distended neck veins; weak, spontaneous cough; sounds of congestion, but no sputum produced; bilateral dull percussion notes, crackles, and rhonchi; Vital signs: BP 180/120, HR 130, RR 26, T 37.8° C (100° F); hemodynamics: increased CVP, RAP, $\overline{PA}$, RVSWI, and PVR; all other hemodynamic values, including PCWP, normal; oxygenation indices: increased $\dot{Q}s/\dot{Q}T$, and O_2ER and decreased DO_2 and $S\overline{v}O_2$; $\dot{V}O_2$ and $C(a - \overline{v})O_2$ normal; ABGs; pH 7.57, $PaCO_2$ 49, HCO_3^- 40, PaO_2 43; SpO_2 76%

Response 2–cont'd

A: • Severe kyphoscoliosis (history, physical exam, ABGs, CXR)
   • Increased work of breathing, worsening (increased blood pressure, heart rate, and respiratory rate)
   • Excessive bronchial secretions (rhonchi, congested cough)
   • Atelectasis and consolidation (previous CXR)
   • Acute alveolar hyperventilation superimposed on chronic ventilatory failure with moderate-to-severe hypoxemia (ABGs and history)
      Continued critically ill status, but chances of avoiding ventilatory failure improving

P: Up-regulate Oxygen Therapy Protocol (e.g., HAFOE at 0.35). Up-regulate Bronchial Hygiene Therapy Protocol (e.g., CPT and PD qid). Up-regulate Aerosolized Medication Protocol (e.g., increase in IPPB med. nebs. to q2h). Contact physician regarding possible ventilatory failure. Discuss therapeutic bronchoscopy with physician. Continue to keep mechanical ventilator on standby. Monitor and reevaluate in 30 minutes.

Response 3

S: "I feel so much better. I finally have enough wind to eat some food."

O: Pale and cyanotic appearance; cough: strong, small amount of white sputum; vital signs: BP 140/85, HR 83, RR 14, T normal; crackles, rhonchi, and dull percussion notes over both lung fields; rhonchi improving; hemodynamic and oxygenation indices improving, but still an elevated CVP, RAP, $\overline{PA}$, RVSWI, and PVR and still an increased $\dot{Q}s/\dot{Q}t$ and O_2ER and a decreased Do_2 and $S\overline{v}o_2$; CXR: improvement of the bilateral pneumonia and atelectasis; ABGs; pH 7.45, $Paco_2$ 73, HCO_3^- 48, Pao_2 68; Spo_2 93%

A: • Generally improved respiratory status (history, CXR, hemodynamic and oxygenation indices, ABGs)
   • Significant improvement in problem with excessive bronchial secretions (rhonchi, cough)
   • Improvement in atelectasis and consolidation (CXR)
   • Chronic ventilatory failure with mild hypoxemia (ABGs)
      Current ABGs likely close to patient's normal ABGs

P: Down-regulate Oxygen Therapy, Bronchial Hygiene Therapy, and Aerosolized Medication Protocols. Continue to monitor and reevaluate (e.g., ABGs on reduced Fio_2). Recommend pulmonary rehabilitation and patient and family education (e.g., possibly rocking bed, positive expiratory pressure [PEP], or cuirass respiratory ventilation).

DISCUSSION

Care of the patient with symptomatic advanced kyphoscoliosis consists of (1) treatment of the conditions that can complicate it (e.g., bronchitis, pneumonia, atelectasis, pleural effusion) and (2) treatment of the underlying condition itself.

With respect to the issue of long-term ventilatory support, the direct treatment of respiratory pump failure as it occurs in kyphoscoliotic lung disease is limited by whether the patient is willing to spend the last months or years of life on a ventilator.

Initial evaluation of this patient suggests that infection is present because of the yellow sputum and recent history. The initial chest x-ray also suggests this. Clearly respiratory failure is impending, and the therapist's desire to cautiously oxygenate the patient, give bronchial hygiene and mucolytic aerosols, and to be prepared for ventilator support are all appropriate. The patient's secondary polycythemia and cor pulmonale should improve as overall oxygenation improves, although this improvement may take some time. The patient's hypertension may reflect CO_2 retention, which must be monitored carefully. The digital clubbing and cor pulmonale itself suggest that the hypoxemia is long standing.

At the time of the **second assessment** the patient still demonstrates signs of atelectasis or pneumonia despite vigorous bronchial hygiene therapy. For example, these conditions were verified by the continued observation of the high pulse and respiratory rate, dull percussion notes, acute alveolar hyperventilation, **atelectasis** on the chest x-ray, and poor response to oxygen therapy (see Fig. 1-8).

Atelectasis is often refractory to oxygen therapy, suggesting that therapeutic bronchoscopy might be worthwhile. Although the outlook seems dismal at this point, many clinicians find that vigorous treatment of the complicating factors (in this case hypertension and atelectasis or pneumonia) often carries the day and that the patient does recover, despite early predictions to the contrary.

Recovery indeed seems to be the case at the time of the **last assessment.** The patient is still retaining CO_2. Indeed the $Paco_2$ is higher than it was on admission. However, the reader should know that the high $Paco_2$ is close to the patient's normal level. In fact, according to the pH (normal but on the alkalotic side of normal) the patient's usual $Paco_2$ is most likely somewhat higher than this last assessment value.

Comparison with baseline values would be appropriate at this time, and consideration of cuirass ventilation, a rocking bed, or NIPPV to assist nocturnal ventilation may be in order. Oxygenation easily can be assessed by oximetry at home. This case is an excellent example of the value of hemodynamic monitoring (specifically the normal PCWP) in differentiating left-sided from right-sided cardiac failure.

Chapter 17   Pneumoconiosis

Response 1

S: "This is the worst my breathing has ever been."

O: Vital signs: BP 180/96, HR 108, RR 32, T 38.3° C (100.8° F); weak appearance; skin: cyanotic, damp, and clammy; distended neck veins and digital clubbing; cough: frequent, weak, moderate amount of thick, whitish yellow secretions; peripheral edema (3+) of ankles and feet. Bilateral dull percussion notes in lung bases. Over both lungs: wheezing, rhonchi, and crackles; pleural friction rub over right middle lobe between sixth and seventh ribs, between anterior axillary line and midaxillary line; CXR: "ground-glass" appearance in lower lobes; calcified pleural plaques in right and left lower pleural spaces; consolidation in right middle lung lobe; right heart enlargement; ABGs (1.5 L/min O_2 by nasal cannula): pH 7.56, $PaCO_2$ 51, HCO_3^- 38, PaO_2 47

A: • Respiratory distress (general appearance, vital signs, ABGs)
  • Pulmonary fibrosis (history, diagnosis of asbestosis, CXR)
  • Alveolar consolidation in right middle lobe (CXR)
  • Pleurisy (asbestosis or pneumonitis) in right middle lobe (pleural friction rub)
  • Excessive bronchial secretions (rhonchi, sputum production)
    Infection likely (yellow sputum)
  • Bronchospasm (wheezing)
    Wheezing possibly caused by bronchial secretions
  • Acute alveolar hyperventilation superimposed on chronic ventilatory failure with moderate-to-severe hypoxemia (history, ABGs)
    Possible impending ventilatory failure (ABGs)

P: Begin Oxygen Therapy Protocol (e.g., HAFOE at FIO_2 0.28) and Aerosolized Medication Protocol (e.g., 2 cc premixed albuterol qid), followed by Bronchial Hygiene Therapy Protocol (e.g., C&DB q4h; obtaining sputum for Gram's stain and culture). Initiate Hyperinflation Therapy Protocol (e.g., incentive spirometry followed by C&DB). Monitor with alarming pulse oximeter set at 85% SpO_2.

Response 2

S: N/A (patient too dyspneic to reply)

O: Condition unstable; cough: frequent, weak, productive of thick, white and yellow secretions; skin: cyanotic, pale, cool, and damp; distended neck veins and peripheral edema, but improving; vital signs: BP 192/108, HR 113, RR 34, T 38° C (100.4° F); dull percussion notes over both lung bases; wheezing, rhonchi, and crackles throughout both lungs; pleural friction rub over right middle lobe between sixth and seventh ribs, between anterior axillary line and midaxillary line; ABGs: pH 7.57, $PaCO_2$ 47, HCO_3^- 36, PaO_2 40; SpO_2 77%

Continued

Response 2—cont'd

A: • Continued respiratory distress (general appearance, vital signs, ABGs)
   • Pulmonary fibrosis in lower lobes (history, diagnosis of asbestosis, recent CXR)
   • Alveolar consolidation in right middle lobe (CXR, pneumonia)
   • Pleurisy or pneumonia that has extended into pleural space over right middle lobe (pleural friction rub)
   • Excessive bronchial secretions (rhonchi, sputum production)
     Infection likely (yellow sputum)
   • Bronchospasm (wheezing)
     Wheezing not improving in response to bronchodilator treatment
     Wheezing possibly caused by bronchial secretions
   • Acute alveolar hyperventilation superimposed on chronic ventilatory failure with severe hypoxemia, worsening (history, ABGs)
     Impending ventilatory failure (ABGs)

P: Up-regulate oxygen therapy per protocol (e.g., HAFOE at F_{IO_2} 0.40). Continue Bronchial Hygiene Therapy and Aerosolized Medication Protocols (e.g., adding intensive nasotracheal suctioning q2h and 2 cc acetyl-cysteine to the premix albuterol). Continue Hyperinflation Therapy Protocol (e.g., continuing to coach and monitor incentive spirometry; if FVC falls below 15 cc/kg, substituting IPPB with previously discussed aerosolized medications while awake). Continue to monitor closely.

Response 3

S: N/A (patient intubated on ventilator)

O: Vital signs: BP 135/90 on vasopressor, HR 84, T 38.3° C (100.8° F); frequent premature ventricular contractions; skin: pale, cyanotic, and clammy; distended neck veins; peripheral edema of ankles and feet; dull percussion notes over lung bases; wheezing, rhonchi, and crackles throughout both lungs; thick, greenish-yellow sputum frequently suctioned; pleural friction rub over right middle lung lobe between sixth and seventh ribs and between anterior axillary line and midaxillary line; hemodynamic indices: elevated CVP, RAP, $\overline{PA}$, RVSWI, and PVR; ABGs: pH 7.53, $Paco_2$ 56, HCO_3^- 38, Pao_2 246; Spo_2 98%

A: • Pulmonary fibrosis, lower lung lobes (history, diagnosis of asbestosis, recent CXR)
   • Alveolar consolidation, right middle lobe (recent CXR showing pneumonia)
   • Pneumonia possibly extended into pleural space over right middle lobe (pleural friction rub)
   • Excessive bronchial secretions (rhonchi, sputum production)
     Infection likely (greenish-yellow sputum, possible new organism)
     Bronchospasm possible (wheezing)
     Wheezing not improving in response to bronchodilator treatment
     Wheezing possibly caused by bronchial secretions
   • Acute alveolar hyperventilation superimposed on chronic ventilatory failure and overly corrected hypoxemia (ABGs)
     Overventilation (mechanical) and overoxygenation

P: Down-regulate Oxygen Therapy Protocol (e.g., reduction of F_{IO_2} to 0.50). Down-regulate Mechanical Ventilation Protocol (e.g., decreasing tidal volume or rate). Continue bronchial hygiene therapy and aerosolized medication per protocol. Continue Hyperinflation Therapy Protocol (depending on mean airway pressure). Continue to closely monitor and reevaluate.

DISCUSSION

The admitting history reveals that the patient has been diagnosed with moderate pneumoconiosis (probable asbestosis) and that he has been a heavy smoker for more than 40 years. Not surprisingly, pulmonary function tests in the past have shown mild-to-moderate combined obstructive and restrictive pulmonary disorders.

What is new is the history suggesting congestive heart failure and the arterial blood gases on his discharge from the hospital 10 months before this admission, which demonstrated chronic ventilatory failure. The patient's recent fever and cough before his emergency room admission suggest an infectious cause for his symptoms. His cyanosis, neck-vein distention, and digital clubbing suggest chronic hypoxemia. The sputum secretions confirm that infection may indeed be present and that the assessing therapist's desire to obtain a sputum culture is appropriate. The pleural rub demonstrated by this patient could be related to his asbestosis or to a pneumonic infiltrate extending to the pleural surface.

In the **initial assessment** the patient's severe hypertension and his fever should be noted. Both deserve vigorous therapy if his pulmonary function is to improve at all. The patient's severe hypoxemia reflects **alveolar-capillary membrane thickening** (see Fig. 1-10) and **pneumonic consolidation** (see Fig. 1-9). The latter is possibly treatable, and therapy is appropriately directed to reduction of intrapulmonary shunting. Note that the pulmonary capillary wedge pressure (PCWP) was not measured in the first assessments. Such measurements may have identified an element of *left* ventricular failure in this hypertensive patient as well. The patient is hyperventilating with respect to his earlier outpatient blood gases. This assessment should record the patient's underlying pulmonary conditions (chronic pulmonary fibrosis, bronchitis, and congestive heart failure) but should really zero in on the treatable issues, specifically the pulmonary infection, as suggested by the sputum and chest x-ray film.

At the time of the **second evaluation** the patient's hypoxemia has worsened despite oxygen therapy. If not already being used, Venturi oxygen mask (HAFOE) therapy is indicated here, and additional mucolytics and endobronchial suctioning also may be indicated. The trial of hyperinflation therapy would have to be made carefully, given the patient's known airway obstruction. A trial of diuretic therapy to reduce the fluid retention may have been ordered by the physician. The therapist's opinion that the wheezing might have been caused by bronchial secretions, rather than by out-and-out bronchospasm, very possibly is correct. However, the distinction is academic because both aerosolized medication therapy and mucolytics should be used in this setting.

The **last assessment** reveals ventricular arrhythmias. The change in the patient's sputum color from thick and white to greenish-yellow suggests superinfection with another organism, and reculture of the sputum is appropriate. The patient is hyperoxygenated, and the F_{IO_2} should be reduced appropriately. Ventilator parameters should be adjusted to provide good pulmonary expansion while avoiding high mean airway pressures.

Despite all that was done for this patient, he died as a result of left congestive heart failure and pneumonia complicating his pulmonary asbestosis.

Chapter 18   Cancer of the Lungs

Response 1

S: "I've coughed up a cup of sputum since breakfast."

O: Vital signs: BP 155/85, HR 90, RR 22, T normal; perspiration and weak and cyanotic appearance; voice hoarse-sounding; weak cough; large amounts of blood-streaked sputum; dull percussion notes over left lower lobe; rhonchi, wheezing, and crackles throughout both lung fields; recent PFT: restrictive and obstructive pulmonary disorder; CT scan and CXR: 2- to 5-cm masses in right and left mediastinum in hilar regions and atelectasis of left lower lobe; bronchoscopy: protruding tumors in both left and right large airways, mucus plugging; biopsy; squamous cell bronchogenic carcinoma; ABGs (2 L/min O_2 by nasal cannula): pH 7.51, $PaCO_2$ 29, HCO_3^- 22, PaO_2 66; SpO_2 92%

A: • Bronchogenic carcinoma (CT scan and biopsy)
 • Respiratory distress (vital signs, ABGs)
 • Excessive bloody bronchial secretions (sputum, rhonchi)
   Mucus plugging likely (bronchoscopy)
 • Poor ability to mobilize secretions (weak cough)
 • Atelectasis of left lower lobe (CXR)
 • Acute alveolar hyperventilation with mild hypoxemia (ABGs)

P: Initiate Oxygen Therapy Protocol (e.g., 4 L nasal cannula and titration by oximetry). Also begin Aerosolized Medication Protocol (e.g., 0.5 cc albuterol in 2 cc 10% acetylcysteine q6h), followed by Bronchial Hygiene Therapy Protocol (e.g., C&DB). Begin Hyperinflation Therapy Protocol (e.g., incentive spirometry q2h and prn). Closely monitor and reevaluate.

Response 2

S: "I'm still not breathing very well."

O: Vital signs: BP 166/90, HR 95, RR 28, T normal; vomiting over past 10 hours; cyanosis, tiredness and dampness from perspiration; cough: weak and productive of moderately thick, clear and white sputum; dull percussion notes over both right and left lower lobes; rhonchi, wheezing, and crackles over both lung fields; ABGs: pH 7.55, $PaCO_2$ 25, HCO_3^- 20, PaO_2 53, SpO_2 88%

A: • Bronchogenic carcinoma (previous CT scan and biopsy)
 • Trouble tolerating chemotherapy well (excessive vomiting)
 • Continued respiratory distress
 • Excessive bronchial secretions (sputum, rhonchi)
   Mucus plugging still likely (previous bronchoscopy, secretions becoming thicker)
 • Poor ability to mobilize secretions (weak cough)
 • Atelectasis of left lower lobes; atelectasis likely in right lower lobe now (CXR, dull percussion notes)
 • Acute alveolar hyperventilation with moderate hypoxemia, worsening (ABGs)
   Possible impending ventilatory failure

Response 2–cont'd

P: Up-regulate Oxygen Therapy Protocol (e.g., oxygen mask). Up-regulate Aerosolized Medication Protocol (e.g., increasing treatment frequency to q3h). Up-regulate Bronchial Hygiene Therapy Protocol (e.g., CPT and PD q3h). Up-regulate Hyperinflation Therapy Protocol (e.g., changing incentive spirometry to IPPB). Contact physician about possible ventilatory failure. Discuss therapeutic bronchoscopy. Closely monitor and reevaluate.

Response 3

S: N/A (patient comatose)

O: Unresponsive; pale, cyanotic, and perspiring appearance; no cough noted; rhonchi heard without stethoscope; vital signs: BP 170/105, HR 110, RR 11 and shallow, T normal; rhonchi, wheezing, and crackles over both lung fields; ABGs: pH 7.28, $PaCO_2$ 63, HCO_3^- 27, PaO_2 66; SpO_2 90%

A: • Bronchogenic carcinoma (previous CT scan and biopsy)
   • Excessive bronchial secretions (rhonchi)
       Mucus plugging still likely (previous bronchoscopy, rhonchi)
   • Poor ability to mobilize secretions (no cough)
   • Atelectasis (history)
   • Acute ventilatory failure with moderate hypoxemia (ABGs)

P: Contact physician about acute ventilatory failure and discuss code status. Up-regulate oxygen therapy, bronchial hygiene therapy, and aerosolized medication therapy per respective protocols. Monitor and reevaluate.

DISCUSSION

This case demonstrates the few specific treatments that a respiratory care practitioner can bring to the care of patients with lung cancer. Specifically, it illustrates that most of the patients have concomitant obstructive pulmonary disease with a need for good bronchial hygiene therapy. The patient's comfort must be kept in mind at all times.

The **first assessment** is performed soon after bronchoscopy, and a diagnosis had been made previously. The patient's blood-stained sputum may reflect the primary tumor or, more likely, bleeding from the bronchoscopy sites. The practitioner must monitor this sputum as the day goes along. No improvement in the patient's wheezing can be expected if an endobronchial tumor is the cause, but it may improve if obstructive pulmonary disease (from cigarette smoking) is the causative factor.

The rhonchi, wheezing, and crackles indicate the need for vigorous bronchial hygiene therapy. The **atelectasis** in the left lower lobe suggests that a trial of careful hyperinflation therapy is in order (see Fig. 1-8). The ABGs drawn on 2 L/min O_2 show moderate hypoxemia, despite alveolar hyperventilation. A trial of oxygen by Venturi mask (or nonrebreathing mask) would be helpful. The patient's anxiety may be alleviated with appropriate treatment of the hypoxemia.

The **second assessment** reveals that the patient may have developed atelectasis in both the right and left lower lobes (recalling where the tumor masses were noted previously). This case may be a setting in which therapeutic bronchoscopy or laser-assisted endobronchial resection of the tumor masses may be helpful. The patient continues to be hypoxemic, despite alveolar hyperventilation. A higher F_{IO_2} (through a Venturi oxygen mask) may be indicated. Vigorous suctioning should be done. Ordering at least one cycle of ventilator support for such a patient would not be surprising, given that the patient just recently received radiation and chemotherapy. His wishes in this respect should be checked against his living will or durable power of attorney for health care, if such a document exists.

The **last assessment** indicates that the patient did not elect this type of therapy and that he is now slipping into acute ventilatory failure. All health-care personnel have agreed that the patient is close to death. The practitioner may be excused for not suggesting the use of chest physical therapy and postural drainage at this time because of the patient's wishes. Aerosolized morphine is now being used to relieve dyspnea in terminally ill cancer patients. If, however, aggressive therapy were still in order, formal evaluation and treatment of superimposed atelectasis or pneumonia, or both, would be in order.

Chapter 19   *Adult Respiratory Distress Syndrome*

Response 1

S: "I cannot move very well, and I am becoming short of breath."

O: Vital signs: BP 125/78, HR 93, RR 21, T normal; skin: pale; no cough; nonproductive voluntary cough; tenderness over anterior chest; bilateral lung fields: dull percussion notes, bronchial breath sounds; SpO_2 95%; ABGs (3 L/min O_2 by nasal cannula): pH 7.51, $PaCO_2$ 29, HCO_3^- 22, PaO_2 68, CXR: bilateral "ground-glass" infiltrates worsening

A: • Increased work of breathing (vital signs, ABGs)
  • Increased lung infiltrates: possible atelectasis or consolidation? Possible ARDS? Fat emboli? (CXR, chest assessment findings)
  • Acute alveolar hyperventilation with mild hypoxemia (ABGs)

P: Initiate Hyperinflation Therapy Protocol (e.g., incentive spirometry with therapist qh until 2200; then q2h). Begin Oxygen Therapy Protocol (e.g., HAFOE mask at FIO_2 0.4). Monitor and reevaluate (e.g., in 30 to 60 minutes with ABG).

Response 2

S: "I'm feeling worse."

O: Vital signs: RR 30, BP 165/95, HR 110, T 38.8° C (101.8° F); tender anterior chest; bronchial breath sounds and crackles bilaterally; SpO_2 75%; ABGs: pH 7.56, $PaCO_2$ 24, HCO_3^- 18, PaO_2 35

A: • Continued increased work of breathing (vital signs, ABGs)
  • Worsening of atelectasis or pneumonia (chest assessment, bronchial breath sounds and crackles)
  • Acute alveolar hyperventilation with moderate hypoxemia (ABGs)
  • Impending acute ventilatory failure (ABGs)

P: Contact physician regarding impending ventilatory failure. Up-regulate Oxygen Therapy Protocol (e.g., partial rebreathing mask). Up-regulate Hyperinflation Therapy Protocol (e.g., changing incentive spirometry to IPPB or trial of nasal CPAP at 10 cm H_2O). Monitor and reevaluate (e.g., 1 hour).

Response 3

S: N/A (patient responsive)

O: Vital signs: RR 18, BP 170/97, HR 150, T 37.8° C (100° F); skin: cyanotic; bronchial breath sounds and crackles bilaterally; SpO_2 69%; ABGs: pH 7.31, $PaCO_2$ 48, HCO_3^- 22, PaO_2 31; CXR: increased infiltrates bilaterally

A: • Worsening of interstitial lung process: ARDS or atelectasis versus pneumonia (chest assessment, CXR)
    • Acute ventilatory failure with moderate hypoxemia (ABGs)

P: Contact physician regarding acute ventilatory failure stat. Prepare for immediate intubation and mechanical ventilation. Continue hyperinflation therapy with PEEP per Mechanical Ventilation Protocol. Continue Oxygen Therapy Protocol. Monitor and reevaluate closely.

DISCUSSION

Multiple trauma (including chest wall trauma) in a patient should in itself constitute notification to the therapist that his expertise will be needed. In this patient, who is hypotensive and has fractured teeth along with multiple bone fractures, three diagnoses should immediately come to mind: (1) the patient's potential for developing adult respiratory distress syndrome (ARDS), (2) the possibility that dental fragments were aspirated, causing obstructive pneumonia or atelectasis, and (3) fat emboli, which could complicate an already serious situation. A diagnosis of possible pulmonary contusion also would be in order, given the history of chest trauma, the short interval between the injury and the abnormal chest x-ray, and that the x-ray abnormalities seemed out of proportion to the ABGs as measured. The patient's tachypnea, dyspnea, tachycardia, and hypoxemia all reflect the effects of the pathophysiologic abnormalities seen with **atelectasis** (see Fig. 1-8) and/or **increased alveolar-capillary thickening**–diffusion blockade (see Fig. 1-10).

At the time of the **first evaluation** the development of progressive hypoxemia, "ground-glass" infiltrates in the chest film, and increasing dyspnea 24 hours or so after multiple trauma are almost pathognomonic of ARDS. Examination and assessment have determined that despite his frontal chest injury, the patient does *not* have a flail chest. The probability that the patient will require intubation and mechanical ventilation with positive end-expiratory pressure (PEEP) or inverse ratio ventilation is high.

A trial of hyperinflation therapy (e.g., with mask continuous positive airway pressure [CPAP]) is indicated in this setting but is often not successful because of patient intolerance. Preparation should be made for intubation and mechanical ventilation in case the pulmonary function decreases any further. Initially the patient should be placed on mask oxygen therapy to improve oxygenation and supply him with a known FIO_2 so that the alveolar-arterial oxygen gradient can be calculated (knowing that the patient will likely be refractory, to some degree, to oxygen therapy). Hyperinflation therapy with incentive spirometry or intermittent positive-pressure breathing (IPPB) is indicated but may not be well tolerated because of chest pain.

Prompt (30 to 60 minutes) reevaluation with repeat arterial blood gas (ABG) measurement is indicated.

At the time of the **second evaluation** 3 days after surgery, the patient has not improved and, indeed, is feeling worse. He is cyanotic and tachypneic, and his ABG values show profound deterioration, with a PaO_2 of 35 mm Hg and a $PaCO_2$ of 24 mm Hg. An attempt may be made at this point to increase his hyperinflation therapy with a positive expiratory pressure (PEP) mask or CPAP, but it will probably be futile. If the patient is not on an FIO_2 of 1.0, he should be. Review of the chest film is mandatory because a complicating problem such as a pneumothorax could theoretically have occurred, or a large pleural effusion could have developed. If the reader is ready to intubate the patient at this point, it is justified.

The **last evaluation** occurs 30 minutes after the second one. The patient is unresponsive. His auscultatory findings have not changed, but his blood gases have deteriorated still further. If protocol allows, the patient should be intubated immediately. If not, the attending physician should be called to request intubation and the immediate start of mechanical ventilation and PEEP.

With this aggressive therapy the patient gradually improved. He remained on a mechanical ventilator for 14 days and then spent an additional 1 month recovering in the hospital. During this recovery another pulmonary complication in the form of an acute pulmonary embolus developed. He recovered and was discharged eventually to his home on supplemental oxygen and was subsequently lost to follow-up care.

Recent studies have suggested that lung function never completely returns to normal after a significant bout of ARDS. These effects, however, may be minimal; for example, exercise may produce mild oxygen desaturation as an effect of lung tissue remodeling.

KEY POINT ANSWERS

For ARDS (DRG* 99/100)

1. Basic Concept Formation
   a. *Trauma* is associated with flail chest, pulmonary contusion, pulmonary emboli, pneumothorax, and adult respiratory distress syndrome (ARDS)
   b. *Infection* is associated with pneumonia, empyema, and ARDS.
   c. *Yes.*
2. Database Formation
   a. First described clearly in 1967, ARDS has been associated with the following conditions:
      1. Sepsis or sepsis syndrome (systemic inflammatory response syndrome [SIRS])
      2. Gastric aspiration
      3. Trauma
      4. Heroin and other drug overdose
      5. Multiple transfusions
      6. Fat emboli
      7. Chemical or smoke inhalation
      8. Burns
      9. Disseminated intravascular coagulation (DIC)
      10. Viral pneumonia
      11. Pancreatitis
      12. Drug reactions
      13. Near drowning
   b. *Systemic inflammatory response syndrome (SIRS)* has been identified recently by the presence of two or more of the following criteria:
      1. Body *temperature* greater than 38° C (100.4° F) or less than 36° C (98.6° F)
      2. *Heart rate* greater than 90 beats per minute
      3. *Tachypnea:* Respiratory rate greater than 20 breaths per minute or $Paco_2$ less than 32 mm Hg
      4. Alterations in white blood cell count (WBC): greater than 12,000/mm^3 or less than 4,000/mm^3 or the presence of greater than 10% immature neutrophils (bands)

      SIRS is an evolving process, involving multiple organ failure (MOF) at sites remote from the initial insult. ARDS is but one expression of SIRS/MOF.
   c. ARDS produces acute *inflammation of the alveolar-capillary membrane*† *with hyaline membrane formation, atelectasis,* and an element of *alveolar consolidation. Pulmonary hypertension and right-sided heart failure* also may occur.
   d. After injury to the pulmonary capillary endothelium or the alveolar epithelium, *high-permeability pulmonary edema* (HPPE) occurs. (1) The chest x-ray film reveals diffuse, bilateral "ground-glass" infiltrates, (2) extravascular water increases, and (3) *static lung compliance falls.* The pulmonary capillary end-diastolic ("wedge") pressure (PCWP) is normal. *Severe, oxygen-resistant hypoxemia* (shunt physiology) develops.
   e. The goals of therapy are to *treat hypoxemia, stabilize alveolar size, and treat respiratory failure.*

---

*DRG, Diagnosis-related group.
†See color plate 20 in Des Jardins T, Burton GG: Clinical manifestations and assessment of respiratory disease, ed 4, St Louis, 2002, Mosby.

f. Treatment of ARDS is supportive and consists of *oxygen therapy, mechanical ventilation, and positive end-expiratory pressure (PEEP)*. Permissive hypercapnia also is used to limit pulmonary barotrauma. The use of *aerosolized surfactant* is undergoing evaluation. This substance is reduced in individuals with ARDS, as it is in those with the neonatal respiratory distress syndrome (IRDS/NRDS).

Protocol	Expected Outcomes	Possible Adverse Effects	Monitors
Oxygen Therapy (see Protocol 1-1)	Improved hypoxemia	Pulmonary oxygen toxicity	ECG, SpO_2, ABGs
PEEP	Improved static compliance, hypoxemia	Barotrauma	SpO_2, static compliance, ABGs, ventilator graphics
Mechanical ventilation	Improved PaO_2, $PaCO_2$	Barotrauma	ECG, SpO_2, static compliance, ABGs, ventilator graphics

3. Assessment
   a. *Yes.* He had modest tachycardia and tachypnea, bilateral "ground-glass" pulmonary infiltrates, and definite hypoxemia on 3 L/minute oxygen, despite alveolar hyperventilation. What was earlier thought to be a pulmonary contusion clearly progressed.
   b. *Yes.* He suffered extensive trauma to multiple bones and organs, and surgery was prolonged.
   c. *Yes.* He demonstrated the effects of *relative shunt physiology, reduced lung compliance, and alveolar inflammation*, all of which should have been clear by the time of the *second assessment*.
   d. ARDS is a *severe disease* by definition.
   e. Pulmonary *infectious complications* account for most ARDS deaths. During the course of the illness presented in these three scenarios, the patient had not yet developed them. He eventually did develop *pulmonary embolic disease*, which is a known complication of trauma and prolonged immobilization. He never did develop *chronic ventilatory failure*, which is seen in a small number of ARDS patients.
4. Application
   a. Oxygen therapy *was* indicated from the start because of the patient's *hypoxemia*.
   b. Monitoring *was* indicated because of the patient's *hypoxemia and overall status*.
   c. Hyperinflation therapy *was* indicated to *stabilize the atelectasis-prone alveoli*.
5. Evaluation
   a. Following are the expected results of each aspect of therapy selected:
      1. *Satisfactory oxygenation* (SaO_2, 90%) should result from use of the Oxygen Therapy Protocol.
      2. *Adequate gas exchange* should occur when mechanical ventilation or PEEP is instituted. An attempt should be made to keep mean airway pressures as low as possible; *permissive hypercapnia* may be necessary.
   b. See *monitors* listed in answer 2.f.
   c. *Oxygen therapy* as listed can be carried up to an FIO_2 of 1.0. *Mask CPAP* can be tried in the short term but is generally poorly tolerated because of aerophagia and pressure discomfort from the mask. Unfortunately, mechanical ventilation or PEEP therapy, with its attendant costs and hazards, is almost always necessary in these patients. *Continued*

d. The risks of mechanical ventilation therapy are *barotrauma* and *oxygen toxicity* from prolonged high-concentration oxygen therapy.

e. If the patient improves, the ventilator FIO_2 should be reduced first; then the PEEP should be tapered; then pressure support ventilation (PSV) weaning should be started.

f. If the patient does not improve on high PEEP or high FIO_2 therapy, specialized centers may try extracorporeal membrane oxygenation *(ECMO)* or *nitrous oxide ventilation.*

6. Boundary Awareness

a. *Increasing pulmonary infiltrates* on chest x-ray films, a *widening alveolar-arterial oxygen gradient,* and *falling static pulmonary compliance are signs of worsening* in ARDS.

b. You should probably consult a supervisor at the time of the *first assessment* because these patients progress downhill rapidly in the early stages of ARDS.

c. You should call the physician by the time of the *second assessment,* when the patient's ARDS is clear.

d. *Serial ABG determinations* document acute ventilatory failure, which was seen at the time of the *third assessment.*

e. *Barotrauma, secondary pulmonary infection, and occasional oxygen toxicity* are all risks of therapy.

Chapter 20   *Chronic Interstitial Lung Disease*

Response 1

S: "I had to stop taking my aerobic class because of shortness of breath."

O: Vital signs: BP 145/90, HR 96, RR 28, T normal; cyanosis, digital clubbing; frequent, dry, nonproductive cough; peripheral edema, distended neck veins, and enlarged and tender liver; pursed-lip breathing; bilateral bronchial breath sounds and crackles; tactile and vocal fremitus over lung bases; PFTs: moderate restrictive and obstructive disorder; 50% reduction in D_{LCO}; CXR: bilateral diffuse interstitial infiltrates and nodular densities in lower lung lobes, air bronchograms, right ventricular cardiomegaly; ABGs (room air): pH 7.53, $Paco_2$ 29, HCO_3^- 21, Pao_2 61

A: • Moderate respiratory distress (history, vital signs, ABGs)
 • Bilateral interstitial infiltrates (CXR) with combined obstructive and restrictive elements (PFTs)
 • Bronchial obstruction, possibly bronchospasm (PFT)
 • Cor pulmonale (CXR)
 • Acute alveolar hyperventilation with mild-to-moderate hypoxemia (ABGs)

P: Initiate Oxygen Therapy per protocol (e.g., 2 L/min by nasal cannula) and trial period of Hyperinflation Therapy Protocol (e.g., incentive spirometry). Begin trial of Aerosolized Medication Protocol (e.g., salmeterol 2 puffs MDI bid). Monitor and reevaluate (e.g., per shift)

Response 2

S: "I'm getting tired of being in the hospital."

O: Appearance weak and tired; cough: frequent, dry; pursed-lip breathing and cyanotic nail beds; vital signs: BP 142/91, HR 90, RR 23, T normal; bilateral bronchial breath sounds and crackles; PEFR: 280 before and after bronchodilator therapy; CXR: bilateral diffuse interstitial infiltrates and nodular densities in lower lobes and air bronchograms; right ventricular cardiomegaly; histology report: sarcoidosis; gallium scan positive; ABGs: pH 7.48, $Paco_2$ 32, HCO_3^- 23, Pao_2 67; Spo_2 94%

A: • Moderate respiratory distress (general observation, vital signs, ABGs)
 • Bilateral interstitial infiltrates (CXR)
 • Active sarcoidosis (histology report, CXR, gallium scan)
 • Bronchial obstruction (PEFR), probably from sarcoidosis–without reversibility from bronchodilator
 • Acute alveolar hyperventilation with mild hypoxemia (ABGs)

P: Continue oxygenation therapy per protocol. Discontinue hyperinflation and bronchodilator therapies per protocols. (With the confirmation of sarcoidosis, the effectiveness of hyperinflation and bronchodilator therapy is questionable.) Continue to monitor and reevaluate. Ensure that pulmonary rehabilitation and home care personnel see patient.

Response 3

S: "I feel much better."

O: No longer in respiratory distress (on present O_2 setting); cough: frequent, dry, and hacking; pursed-lip breathing and cyanosis; vital signs: BP 133/86, HR 86, RR 15, T normal; bronchial breath sounds bilaterally; CXR: bilateral diffuse interstitial infiltrates and nodular densities; air bronchograms also seen; ABGs (on 3 lpm by nasal cannula): pH 7.44, $Paco_2$ 36, HCO_3^- 23, Pao_2 84; SpO_2 95%

A: • Bilateral interstitial infiltrates (CXR)
  • Sarcoidosis (histology report)
  • Bronchial obstruction (PEFR)
  • Normal acid-base status with corrected hypoxemia (ABGs)
  • Overall clinical improvement

P: Recommend home care oxygenation therapy per protocol. Schedule exercise oxygen titration study. Check pneumococcal and influenza vaccine status.

DISCUSSION

Respiratory care of the patient with chronic interstitial lung disease involves ensurance of adequate oxygenation, reversal or prevention of atelectasis, and treatment of any obstructive component that may be present. At least three interstitial lung diseases have a strong obstructive component: sarcoidosis, cystic fibrosis, and esoinophilic granuloma (histiocystosis X).

The **first assessment** suggests that hypoxemia and cor pulmonale may be complicating the patient's course early in the disease. Her dyspnea, tachypnea, tachycardia, and nonrefractory hypoxemia are consistent with **alveolar-capillary thickening** (see Fig. 1-10). Interestingly, some airway obstruction is picked up on pulmonary function testing, suggesting that a somewhat atypical clinical scenario-airway obstruction and possible **bronchospasm** also may be present in this case (see Fig. 1-11). Oxygen therapy is certainly indicated. While the workup is proceeding, not much more can be done to treat her illness. This patient was undiagnosed when she came to the clinic, and the effects of corticosteroid therapy would take some time before they would be felt.

In the **second assessment** a gallium scan indicates that the patient has cytoactive sarcoidosis, for which corticosteroid therapy might be helpful. The patient is modestly hypoxic, and oxygen therapy should be up-regulated. Neither wheezing nor crackles has improved, even on a rapid-acting bronchodilator. Thus hyperinflation and bronchodilator therapy might safely be discontinued. These therapies were instituted only on a trial basis.

At the time of the **third assessment,** with continued improvement in oxygenation with appropriate oxygen therapy, all that remains is to prepare for discharge of this patient on a simple program of supplemental oxygen therapy, if indicated. An oxygen titration study also is appropriate for this purpose. This patient should be recognized by this time as having chronic lung disease, no matter what her symptom status. Only time will tell how much of her interstitial disease will be helped by oral corticosteroids.

This patient is now at the age at which both pneumococcal vaccine and influenza vaccine should be given. The pneumococcal vaccine can be given at any time of the year and should be repeated every 5 to 10 years in patients with chronic lung disease. Influenza vaccine should be given yearly during the fall months. A note should be added to the patient's chart that this action has been recommended.

That this patient presented with cor pulmonale suggests that a significant amount of parenchymal lung damage already exists and that supplemental oxygen therapy may be needed for a long time, if not for the remainder of the patient's lifetime.

Chapter 21   *Guillain-Barré Syndrome*

Response 1

S: N/A (intubated on ventilator)

O: Vital signs: BP 126/82, HR 68, RR 12 (controlled); afebrile; no spontaneous breaths; CXR: normal; normal breath sounds; ABGs (on $FIO_2 = 0.40$): pH 7.51, $Paco_2$ 29, HCO_3^- 22, Pao_2 204; SpO_2 98%

A: • Acute alveolar hyperventilation with excessive oxygenation (ABGs)
        Inappropriate ventilator settings
        Excessive alveolar ventilation (increased pH and decreased $Paco_2$)
        FIO_2 too high (ABGs)

P: Adjust mechanical ventilator setting (e.g., decreasing tidal volume and FIO_2) according to protocol. Monitor closely and reevaluate.

Response 2

S: N/A

O: Skin color good; crackles and rhonchi over both lung fields; moderate amount of white, clear secretions being suctioned regularly; vital signs: BP 124/83, HR 74, T 37.7° C (99.8° F); CXR: unremarkable; ABGs: pH 7.44, $Paco_2$ 35, HCO_3^- 24, and Pao_2 98; SpO_2 97%

A: • Normal acid-base and oxygenation status on present ventilator settings (ABGs)
        • Excessive sputum accumulation; possible progression to mucus plugging and atelectasis (crackles, rhonchi, white and clear secretions)

P: Begin bronchial hygiene therapy per protocol (e.g., vigorous tracheal suctioning and obtaining of sputum stain and culture). Begin Hyperinflation Therapy Protocol (e.g., 10 cm H_2O PEEP to offset any early development of atelectasis). Monitor and reevaluate (e.g., 4 × per shift).

Response 3

S: N/A

O: Skin color good; crackles and rhonchi over both lung fields improving; small amount of clear secretions suctioned; vital signs: BP 118/79, HR 68, T normal; no spontaneous respirations; CXR: normal; ABGs: pH 7.42, $PaCO_2$ 37, HCO_3^- 24, PaO_2 97; SpO_2 97%

A: • Normal acid-base and oxygenation status on present ventilator settings (ABGs)
   • Respiratory muscle pump insufficiency (no spontaneous respirations)
   • Secretion control improving (crackles, rhonchi, clear secretions)

P: Continue Ventilator Management Protocol. Continue Bronchial Hygiene Therapy Protocol. Continue Hyperinflation Therapy Protocol. Monitor and reevaluate (e.g., forced expiratory volume in 1 second [FEV_1], negative inspiratory force [NIF] 2 × per shift).

DISCUSSION

Guillain-Barré syndrome is a neuromuscular paralysis that ensues after infection from a neurotropic virus. This patient has a classic history of ascending paralysis and paresthesias and the diagnostic finding of albuminocytologic dissociation in the spinal fluid. In this setting, serial forced vital capacity (FVC) maneuvers must be charted. Once respiratory failure supervenes, intubation and respiratory support on a ventilator become necessary.

By the time of the **first assessment,** early CO_2 retention is present, and given the clinical setting, the patient is appropriately intubated. The initial blood gases show hyperoxia and hyperventilation. An appropriate response would be to adjust the ventilator settings by a reduction in the tidal volume or frequency (or both) and the FIO_2. At the time of this assessment the patient exhibits no evidence of airways obstruction or secretions. Therefore bronchial hygiene therapy is not indicated. Indeed, all that needs to be done is to ensure adequate ventilation and oxygenation on the ventilator.

However, 3 days later, at the time of the **second assessment,** crackles and rhonchi are heard over all lung fields, and the time has come to begin vigorous bronchial hygiene therapy with suctioning and even possibly, therapy with mucolytic agents. Because of the fear of atelectasis, hyperinflation therapy in the form of positive end-expiratory pressure (PEEP) on the ventilator is indicated (see Fig. 1-8). The sputum should be cultured to see whether any infectious organisms are present.

At the time of the **final assessment** (2 days later) the evidence for airway secretions is lessened because the rhonchi no longer can be heard over the lung fields, and the small amount of sputum suctioned appears clear. At this point, downregulation of bronchial hygiene therapy is indicated.

Serial FVC, forced expiratory volume in 1 second (FEV_1), or negative inspiratory force (NIF) measurements should continue to be made until such time as the patient is able to be extubated. Indeed, extubation happened about 3 weeks after the initiation of mechanical ventilation. The patient recovered without incident, and returned to his active lifestyle within a year.

Chapter 22   *Myasthenia Gravis*

Response 1

S: N/A (patient intubated)

O: No spontaneous ventilations; vital signs: BP 132/86, HR 90, RR 10 (controlled), T 38° C (100.5° F); normal breath sounds over right lung; diminished-to-absent breath sounds over left lung; ABGs (on $F_{IO_2} = 0.50$): pH 7.28, Pa_{CO_2} 58, HCO_3^- 24, Pa_{O_2} 52; Sp_{O_2} 80%

A: • Endotracheal tube possibly placed in right main stem bronchi (diminished-to-absent breath sounds over left lung, ABGs)
• Acute ventilatory failure with mild hypoxemia (ABGs)
   Condition likely caused by misplacement of endotracheal tube

P: Notify physician stat. Check CXR. Pull endotracheal tube back, if necessary. Monitor and reevaluate immediately.

Response 2

S: N/A (patient intubated on ventilator)

O: Vital signs: BP 123/75, HR 74, T normal; normal bronchovesicular breath sounds over both lung fields; CXR: endotracheal tube in good position; lungs adequately ventilated; ABGs: pH 7.53, Pa_{CO_2} 27, HCO_3^- 22, Pa_{O_2} 176; Sp_{O_2} 98%

A: • Acute ventilator-induced alveolar hyperventilation with overly corrected hypoxemia (ABGs)

P: Adjust present mechanical ventilation setting per protocol (e.g., decreasing tidal volume). Down-regulate oxygen therapy per protocol. Monitor and reevaluate.

Response 3

S: N/A

O: No improvement seen in muscular paralysis; skin: pale; vital signs: BP 146/88, HR 92, T 37.9° C (100.2° F); large amounts of thick, yellowish sputum; rhonchi over both lung fields; CXR: pneumonia and atelectasis in right lower lobe; ABGs: pH 7.28, Pa_{CO_2} 36, HCO_3^- 17, Pa_{O_2} 41; Sp_{O_2} 69%

Response 3–cont'd

A: • Excessive bronchial secretions (rhonchi, sputum)
Infection likely (yellow sputum, fever, CXR: pneumonia)
  • Metabolic acidosis with moderate-to-severe hypoxemia (ABGs)
Condition likely caused by lactic acid (ABGs)

P: Up-regulate Bronchial Hygiene Therapy Protocol (e.g., med. neb. with 0.5 cc albuterol in 2 cc 10% acetyl-cysteine q4h; therapist to suction patient frequently; sputum culture check in 24 and 48 hours). Perform Hyperinflation Therapy Protocol (e.g., adding 10 cm H_2O PEEP to ventilator settings). Up-regulate Oxygen Therapy Protocol. Monitor closely and reevaluate (e.g., checking ABGs in 30 minutes).

DISCUSSION

Like the patient with Guillain-Barré syndrome, this case of myasthenia gravis provides yet another chance to discuss ventilatory pump failure secondary to neuromuscular disease. The presentation of this patient with diplopia, dysphagia, and progressive muscle weakness is classic for this condition. The positive Tensilon test noted in the history is necessary for a final diagnosis. Also important to note is that aspiration of gastric contents is not uncommon in these cases.

In the **first assessment** the therapist should recognize that this case is more than simple respiratory pump failure. The reader sees that the patient was intubated recently and that breath sounds no longer are present in the entire left lung (inadvertent right main stem bronchus intubation). The reader should confirm the impression with a chest x-ray and (very quickly) pull the endotracheal tube back and recheck its new placement with another x-ray. At this point, oxygenating the patient is of primary importance. Increasing the FIO_2 to between 0.80 and 1.0 is appropriate. Any attempt to wean the patient at this early junction *should not* proceed.

The **second assessment** should reflect that the patient is improving and is now hyperventilated and hyperoxygenated on the current ventilator settings. The therapist should adjust the ventilator therapy accordingly and begin the process of longitudinal evaluation of forced vital capacity, forced expiratory volume in 1 second, and negative inspiratory force that is appropriate for this condition if weaning is to be accomplished successfully.

The **final assessment** suggests that the patient has taken another downturn. The sputum is now purulent; rhonchi are heard over both lung fields; and a right lower lobe pneumonia or atelectasis has developed. The patient now has an uncompensated metabolic acidemia that needs evaluation.

The therapist should have anticipated this development, obtained appropriate cultures, and if not done before, prophylactically started bronchial hygiene and aerosolized medication therapies with frequent suctioning, percussion and postural drainage, and possibly mucolytics. The metabolic acidemia is out of proportion to the patient's condition as described. The reader may wish to review other possible causes of metabolic acidemia at this time (diabetic ketoacidosis, renal failure, etc.).

Unfortunately the patient's pulmonary condition progressively deteriorated, and she died 3 weeks later.

Chapter 23   Sleep Apnea

Response 1

S: "I'm breathing OK."

O: Weight: >160 kg (355 lb); skin: flushed and cyanotic; distended neck veins and edema of feet and legs (4+) to midcalf; vital signs: BP 194/118, HR 78, RR 22, T normal; oropharyngeal exam typical for obstructive sleep apnea; diminished breath sounds, likely due to obesity; CXR: cor pulmonale; lungs appearing normal; ABGs (on room air): pH 7.54, $PaCO_2$ 48, HCO_3^- 48, PaO_2 52; SpO_2 87%

A: • Obstructive sleep apnea likely (history, cor pulmonale, ABGs, physical appearance)
  • Acute alveolar hyperventilation superimposed on chronic ventilatory failure with moderate hypoxemia (ABGs)
  • Possible impending ventilatory failure

P: Initiate oxygen therapy per protocol. If obstructive sleep apnea is confirmed, start continuous positive airway pressure (CPAP) calibration study. Monitor and reevaluate (e.g., ECG and SpO_2 qh).

Response 2

S: "I'm breathing much better."

O: Recent diagnosis: obstructive sleep apnea—more than 325 periods of obstructive apnea documented during sleep study; short muscular neck; narrow upper airway; obesity; Hct. 51%; Hb 17 g/dl; PFTs: severe restrictive disorder; saw-tooth pattern seen on maximal inspiratory and expiratory flow-volume loops; no longer appearing short of breath; cyanotic appearance but improved; clear but diminished breath sounds; ABGs (on room air): pH 7.38, $PaCO_2$ 82, HCO_3^- 44, PaO_2 66; SpO_2 91%

A: • Obstructive sleep apnea confirmed (history, polysomnographic study, ABGs)
  • Chronic ventilatory failure with mild hypoxemia

P: Continue oxygen therapy per protocol. Request CPAP calibration study. Ensure that patient sleeps in the head-up position and avoids sleeping on his back. Request nutrition service to consult regarding slow weight loss program. Monitor and reevaluate.

DISCUSSION

Although the diagnosis of obstructive sleep apnea is made most frequently in the outpatient setting, recent experience has shown that it often may be diagnosed in the course of an acute hospitalization. In the present case, although the patient was first seen in the emergency room, it soon became clear that he was ill enough to be admitted, and his workup proceeded from there.

In the **first assessment** the therapist must perform a careful examination of the patient's nasopharynx and oropharynx, as well as his chest. The typical anatomy of obstructive sleep apnea is visible. While the patient's polysomnogram and CPAP titration study are in progress, the therapist appropriately ensures the patient's oxygenation (probably by use of a Venturi oxygen mask) to prevent alveolar hypoventilation. In a patient with as classic a case as this, a split night study (half standard polysomnography, half CPAP titration) may be in order.

The patient's neck vein distension, polycythemia, cardiomegaly, and peripheral edema all suggest cor pulmonale. This condition will improve once the patient's overall hypoventilation is treated. Many physicians would go ahead and give the patient a bicarbonate-losing diuretic, watching for worsening of metabolic acidosis while this step is being done. The therapist (in this first assessment) correctly analyzes the situation as being potentially hazardous, and this assessment includes impending ventilatory failure, which is a real possibility.

After the **second assessment** the diagnosis has been made. Pulmonary function tests have shown upper airways obstruction and a restrictive disorder. The therapist ensures that a chest x-ray is taken to rule out any other significant pulmonary condition. None is found. The patient's P_{CO_2}, however, has worsened, and the therapist must make some choices regarding treatment. The therapist elects to have the patient not sleep on his back and to sleep in the head-up position and suggests a nutrition consult because the patient needs to begin a drastic weight-loss program.

At the end of this case the patient still is not markedly improved and awaits the benefits of continuous positive airway pressure (CPAP) therapy. Indeed the CPAP therapy was eventually helpful. The patient had a 9-kg (20-lb) diuresis during the first week of its use, and good oxygenation was achieved with 10 cm H_2O CPAP pressure.

A diagnosis of obstructive sleep apnea often can complicate other primary respiratory disorders, such as chronic obstructive pulmonary disease (COPD), pneumonia, atelectasis, or chest wall deformity. In these settings the care is more complicated and, if anything, should be even more data-driven by careful examination of all subjective and objective data.

Patients with obstructive sleep apnea have a significant risk of cardiovascular and central nervous system morbidity and mortality (myocardial infarctions, arrhythmias, hypertension, and cerebrovascular accidents). Psychiatric effects, such as depression, sleep-related job malperformance, and daytime motor vehicle accidents, also are seen. Current evidence suggests that such patients need *not* experience these effects if the sleep disordered breathing problem is treated effectively. Compliance with CPAP therapy is important, but difficult to measure. Improvement in daytime somnolence is one surrogate for more direct measurements of compliance, such as recording of oximetry in the patient's home. Close clinical monitoring is important if good therapeutic outcomes are to be achieved consistently.

Chapter 24   *Idiopathic (Infant) Respiratory Distress Syndrome*

Response 1

S: N/A

O: Mild respiratory distress: intercostal retractions, nasal flaring, and cyanosis; vital signs: BP 50/20, HR 180, RR 74, T 37.1° C (98.8° F); grunting breath sounds and crackles bilaterally; CXR: mild haziness in lung bases; ABGs (FIO_2 0.40): pH 7.52, $PaCO_2$ 29, HCO_3^- 21, PaO_2 49

A: • Impending infant respiratory distress syndrome (history, CXR)
  • Atelectasis, consolidation, and hyaline membrane formation likely (history, CXR)
  • Acute alveolar hyperventilation with moderate-to-severe hypoxemia (ABGs)

P: Initiate Hyperinflation Therapy Protocol (e.g., nasal CPAP at 5 cm H_2O). Begin Oxygen Therapy Protocol (e.g., FIO_2 at 0.30 via nasal CPAP). Administer exogenous surfactant per protocol. Monitor (e.g., vital signs, breath sounds, and acute changes in color and muscle tone) and evaluate closely. Place infant ventilator on standby.

Response 2

S: N/A

O: Vital signs: RR 30 (ventilator), BP 60/40, HR 184; harsh, bronchial breath sounds and fine crackles bilaterally; CXR: dense, "ground-glass" appearance in both lungs; ABGs (FIO_2 0.60): pH 7.28, $PaCO_2$ 53, HCO_3^- 19, PaO_2 57

A: • Infant respiratory distress syndrome (history, CXR)
  • Worsening of atelectasis, consolidation, and hyaline membrane formation likely (history, CXR)
  • Acute ventilatory failure with severe hypoxemia (ABGs)

P: Continue hyperinflation therapy per Mechanical Ventilation Protocol. Up-regulate oxygenation therapy per Mechanical Ventilation Protocol. Continue the administration of exogenous surfactant per protocol. Constantly monitor ventilator settings to correct acute ventilatory failure (e.g., increasing rate and tidal volume). Monitor and reevaluate closely.

Response 3

S: N/A

O: Vital signs: BP 74/50, HR 120, spontaneous RR 42, T normal; normal vesicular breath sounds; CXR: normal; ABGs: pH 7.42, $PaCO_2$ 37, HCO_3^- 24, PaO_2 162

A: • Appearance that atelectasis, consolidation, and hyaline membrane no longer present (history, CXR)
• Normal ventilatory status with overoxygenation (ABGs)

P: Down-regulate hyperinflation therapy per protocol. Down-regulate oxygen therapy per protocol. Monitor and reevaluate.

DISCUSSION

Infant respiratory distress syndrome (IRDS) is one of the most common complications of prematurity. It can be prevented with aggressive respiratory care. IRDS is referred to often as *hyaline membrane disease* because of the formation of a hyaline membrane inside the alveoli. The problem also is complicated by inadequate surfactant production. The low levels of surfactant in the presence of immature lung tissue produce atelectasis. Hypoxia and pulmonary hypertension develop, which keeps the ductus arteriosus patent and thus allows continuation of fetal circulation after birth. The low Apgar scores on delivery also indicate impending respiratory distress. At this point, hypercapnia and respiratory acidosis occur, which ultimately may prove fatal.

IRDS often is due to lack of prenatal care for the mother. In this case the premature delivery could have been stopped medically with tocolytic drugs, such as terbutaline. That the mother smoked throughout the pregnancy decreased the level of oxygen available to the infant, possibly resulting in the infant's being small for gestational age. The mother's youth in this case also indicates the possibility of a high incidence of complications with the birth.

Initially the low Apgar score indicates that the infant needs constant monitoring. Although cyanosis and crackles are normal signs immediately after delivery, the nasal flaring and intercostal retractions are not. These signs, along with the grunting respirations, indicate impending respiratory failure. The blood pressure is normal, but the infant shows signs of tachypnea and tachycardia, which indicate increased work of breathing. The infant will need an intravenous infusion stat because dehydration and humidification will be additional problems. The infant also should be placed in an open-bed radiant warmer so that a neutral thermal environment is provided immediately.

At the 16-hour assessment the infant is placed on mechanical ventilation because of the clinical findings. Because another dose of surfactant probably has been administered to the child, nasal continuous positive airway pressure (CPAP) could be tried before intubation and placement on the ventilator. Nasal CPAP does not require the passing of a tube through the vocal cords yet aids in the distribution of the surfactant into the distal alveoli.

The **last assessment** shows that the treatment has worked and that the infant continues to improve. The vital signs are all within the normal range; the ABGs indicate that the FIO_2 can continue to be decreased; and the infant can be weaned successfully from mechanical ventilation. The only concern (at this point) is the high PaO_2 because a value less than 100 mm Hg is required to prevent the development of retinopathy of prematurity.

The use of surfactant and the positive end-expiratory pressure (PEEP) or CPAP pressures for aerosol distribution successfully reversed the infant's condition. The short time needed to reverse the IRDS precludes any permanent damage to the lungs, which might have occurred if the infant had remained on the ventilator and developed bronchopulmonary dysplasia.

Chapter 25   *Croup Syndrome*

Response 1

S: N/A (patient crying)

O: Respiratory distress: inspiratory stridor, brassy cough, BP 110/70, HR 160, RR 58, T normal, intercostal and supraclavicular retractions; diminished breath sounds; SpO_2 (O_2 mask) 88%

A: • Croup (moderate to severe) (history, inspiratory stridor)

P: Initiate Oxygen Therapy Protocol. Administer cool mist aerosol treatment and mist tent per protocol. Begin Aerosolized Medication Protocol (e.g., aerosolized racemic epinephrine). Perform throat culture. Monitor closely.

Response 2

S: "I want to go home."

O: Respiratory distress: inspiratory stridor, brassy cough, BP 146/88, HR 155, RR 63, T normal, intercostal and supraclavicular retractions; diminished breath sounds; SpO_2: 90%; lateral neck x-ray film: subglottic haziness

A: • Croup—moderate to severe (history, inspiratory stridor, neck x-ray film)
       • Persistent hypoxemia (SpO_2)

P: Up-regulate oxygen therapy per protocol. Up-regulate cool mist aerosol treatment and mist tent per protocol. Up-regulate aerosolized racemic epinephrine per protocol. Monitor closely.

Response 3

S: Patient nods that he feels better.

O: Inspiratory stridor and supraclavicular retractions no longer present; vital signs: BP 125/80, HR 89, RR 15; normal breath sounds; SpO_2 97%

Continued

Response 3–cont'd

A: • Subglottic edema no longer present

P: Reduce or discontinue oxygen therapy per protocol. Discontinue the aerosol cool mist treatments and cool mist tent. Discontinue aerosolized racemic epinephrine per protocol. Monitor and reevaluate (within 1 hour). If clinical data remains the same, recommend discharge.

DISCUSSION

This case reminds therapists just how sick children can be and how quickly they respond to intelligent therapy. The use of cool mist and decongestant aerosols for this patient, along with appropriate oxygen therapy, clearly prevented the necessity for intubation.

In the **second SOAP evaluation**, therapists who select to recommend intubation cannot be faulted. Many physicians would elect to do so at this juncture unless they feel that persistence and time are often great healers in this condition. Clearly, close monitoring at this juncture is indicated if the child is doing worse.

Finally, the patient was not dyspneic and no longer had stridor or retractions and the apical pulse was 89, respiratory rate 15, blood pressure 125/80, oxygen saturation 97%, and breath sounds normal. This data should be translated directly to the assessment note in the **third SOAP evaluation** because the patient is improving and well on his way to recovery.

Chapter 26   Cystic Fibrosis

Response 1

S: "I've not been this short of breath in a long time."

O: Skin: pale, cyanotic; barrel chest and use of accessory muscles of respiration; digital clubbing; cough frequent and productive; sputum: sweet-smelling, thick, yellow-green; distended neck veins and peripheral edema; vital signs: BP 142/90, HR 108, RR 28, T normal; bilateral hyperresonant percussion notes; diminished breath sounds; crackles and rhonchi; CXR: hyperlucency, flattened diaphragm, and right ventricular enlargement; ABGs (1.5 L/min O_2 by nasal cannula): pH 7.51, $Paco_2$ 58, HCO_3^- 43, Pao_2 66; Spo_2 94%

A: • Respiratory distress (general appearance, vital signs)
  • Excessive tracheobronchial tree secretions (productive cough)
    Infection likely (yellow-green sputum)
  • Hyperinflated alveoli (barrel chest, use of accessory muscles, CXR)
  • Acute alveolar hyperventilation superimposed on chronic ventilatory failure with mild hypoxemia (history, ABGs)
  • Possible impending ventilatory failure
  • Cor pulmonale (distended neck veins, peripheral edema, CXR)

P: Initiate Bronchial Hygiene Therapy Protocol (e.g., C&DB q4h, including a sputum culture). Begin Oxygen Therapy Protocol (e.g., 2 L by nasal cannula). Monitor possible impending ventilatory failure closely (e.g., pulse oximetry, vital signs, ABGs).

Response 2

S: "I can't get enough air to sleep 10 minutes!"

O: Cyanosis and use of accessory muscles of respiration; vital signs: BP 147/95, HR 117, RR 32, T 37° C (98.6° F); cough: frequent, weak, and productive of large amounts of thick, green sputum; *Pseudomonas aeruginosa* cultured; bilateral hyperresonant notes and diminished breath sounds; crackles, rhonchi, and wheezes; Spo_2 92%; ABGs: pH 7.55, $Paco_2$ 54, HCO_3^- 45, Pao_2 57

A: • Continued respiratory distress (general appearance, vital signs, use of accessory muscles)
  • Excessive bronchial secretions (cough, sputum, breath sounds)
    Poor ability to mobilize secretions (weak cough)
  • Acute alveolar hyperventilation superimposed on chronic ventilatory failure with mild-to-moderate hypoxemia (ABGs)
  • Possible impending ventilatory failure

P: Start Aerosolized Medication Protocol (e.g., 0.5 cc albuterol in 2 cc normal saline q4h). Up-regulate bronchial hygiene therapy per protocol (e.g., CPT and trial of bland aerosol q2h). Up-regulate oxygen therapy per protocol (e.g., HAFOE at Fio_2 0.35). Continue to monitor possible impending ventilatory failure closely.

Response 3

S: "I can't get into a comfortable position to breathe."

O: Cyanosis; pursed-lip breathing and use of accessory muscles of respiration; vital signs: BP 145/90, HR 120, RR 22, T 38° C (100.5° F); bilateral hyperresonant percussion notes, crackles, rhonchi, and wheezing; SpO_2 65%; ABGs: pH 7.33, $PaCO_2$ 79, HCO_3^- 41, PaO_2 37

A: • Continued respiratory distress (general appearance, vital signs, use of accessory muscles, pursed-lip breathing)
• Excessive bronchial secretions (cough, sputum, breath sounds)
• Acute ventilatory failure superimposed on chronic ventilatory failure with severe hypoxemia (ABGs, vital signs)

P: Contact physician stat. Consider mechanical ventilation. Up-regulate bronchial hygiene therapy per protocol. Up-regulate oxygen therapy per protocol. Monitor closely.

DISCUSSION

The science of respiratory care has advanced over the years, and the prognosis for patients with this multisystem genetic disorder has improved. In this lifetime at least four therapeutic landmarks can be noted, as follows:

1. Vigorous use of chest physical therapy (percussion and postural drainage)
2. Intermittent treatment of secretions with antibiotics and mucolytic enzymes, such as rhDNase
3. Positive expiratory pressure (PEP) therapy
4. Lung transplantation (when all else fails)

This patient had received at least two of these treatments and was in the hands of caring parents. His own indomitable nature and interest in athletics was clearly helpful in his prolonged survival. Important to note are the circumstances surrounding his *admission,* especially that he had experienced hemoptysis, dyspnea, and weight loss during the period preceding his admission. Note also that he had started smoking cigarettes.

In this case his chief complaints purposely have been buried in the admitting history. The reader should have discerned from it that the patient was coughing productively and had hemoptysis, dyspnea, and weight loss. The recommended therapeutic strategy arises from recognition of these four presenting complaints. Note also that on admission the patient presented with neck vein distension and peripheral edema, suggesting cor pulmonale. If the experience with chronic obstructive pulmonary disease can be translated to patients with cystic fibrosis, this is a bad prognostic sign and one that clearly calls for intensification of the therapeutic regimen.

Note that on the **initial physical examination** no baseline arterial blood gases existed with which to compare his current values. Thus the observation of an elevated $PaCO_2$ should be taken very, very seriously because (at least initially) whether this value is a "chronic" arterial blood gas value is unclear.

At the time of the **second evaluation** the patient clearly is not improving. Bronchial hygiene therapy at this point might consist of increasing chest physical therapy to every hour as tolerated, increasing bronchodilator and mucolytic therapy to every 2 hours, and even consideration of bronchoscopy. If it had not been done earlier, monitoring of electrocardiogram (ECG) and pulse oximetry must be done. A repeat chest x-ray film would not be out of order at this time. In addition, consider that the patient may have an element of metabolic alkalosis, secondary to his malnutrition, diuretic use, or previous nausea and vomiting. The pH is high and is interfering with release of his already-low arterial oxygen to tissues.

The **third assessment** suggests that the patent clearly is deteriorating despite vigorous noninvasive therapy. At this point the patient might be put on a high-concentration Venturi mask, but he probably should be intubated and ventilated. The addition of mechanical ventilation at this time prevents fatigue, allows deep nasal tracheal suctioning, and if necessary facilitates repeat bronchoscopy.

Despite this initial downhill course the patient was placed on a ventilator and slowly improved. Over the next 7 days the patient was extubated. The therapist should note that despite all the "good" things the patient and family did to treat his illness, the patient's initiation of smoking clearly could be a "last-straw" phenomenon. The patient should be placed on a smoking-cessation program. This step is as important for the long-term prognosis as is the skill of the practitioner caring for him during this bout of acute ventilatory failure.

Chapter 27   Near Drowning

Response 1

S: N/A (patient semicomatose, intubated on ventilator)

O: Near-drowning diagnosis; vital signs: BP 137/89, HR 122, RR 12 (controlled), T 32.3° C (90.3° F); crackles and dull percussion notes over right and left lower lobes; CXR: bilateral infiltrates in lower lobes; ABGs (on 50% O_2 and mechanical ventilation): pH 7.23, $Paco_2$ 51, HCO_3^- 19, Pao_2 54; Spo_2 84%

A: • Near drowning (history)
  • Pulmonary edema likely (history, crackles, infiltrates)
  • Acute ventilatory failure with moderate hypoxemia (ABGs)
      Combined metabolic and respiratory acidemia (ABGs)
      Inadequate mechanical ventilation

P: Initiate Hyperinflation Therapy Protocol (e.g., 10 cm H_2O positive end-expiratory pressure [PEEP]). Adjust mechanical ventilator per protocol (e.g., increasing tidal volume or rate to decrease $Paco_2$ and increase pH). Begin Oxygen Therapy Protocol (e.g., increasing Fio_2 to 0.6). Closely monitor and reevaluate.

Response 2

S: N/A (patient intubated on ventilator)

O: Vital signs: BP 125/86, HR 130, T 33.4° C (92.3° F); crackles, rhonchi, and dull percussion notes over right and left lung fields; frothy, white sputum; ABGs: pH 7.53, $Paco_2$ 28, HCO_3^- 21, Pao_2 56; Spo_2 89%

A: • Near drowning (history)
      Possible early ARDS
      Possible gastric aspiration
  • Excessive bronchial secretions (rhonchi, frothy, white sputum, yellow streaks)
  • Acute ventilator-induced alveolar hyperventilation with moderate hypoxemia (ABGs)
      Excessive mechanical ventilation

P: Up-regulate hyperinflation therapy per protocol (e.g., increasing PEEP to 15 cm H_2O. Down-regulate mechanical ventilator per protocol (e.g., decreasing tidal volume or rate to increase $Paco_2$ and decrease pH). Up-regulate oxygen therapy per protocol (e.g., increasing Fio_2 to 1.0). Administer Bronchial Hygiene Therapy Protocol (e.g., CPT qid and suction prn). Closely monitor and reevaluate.

Response 3

S: N/A (patient sedated, intubated on ventilator)

O: Vital signs: BP 100/60, HR 150, T 39.5° C (103° F); cyanotic appearance and cool to touch; pupils: fixed and dilated; crackles and rhonchi over both lung fields worsening; excessive, frothy, pink secretions in endotracheal tube; CXR: fluffy infiltrates consistent with pulmonary edema pattern; ABGs: pH 7.35, $PaCO_2$ 37, HCO_3^- 23, PaO_2 47; SpO_2 80%

A: • Near drowning (history)
   • Pulmonary edema worsening (history, crackles, rhonchi, infiltrates shown in recent CXR)
      Possible ARDS
   • Excessive bronchial secretions (rhonchi, frothy, pinkish-white sputum)
   • Normal acid-base status with moderate-to-severe hypoxemia (ABGs)

P: Up-regulate hyperinflation therapy per protocol (e.g., increasing PEEP to 20 cm H_2O). Up-regulate oxygen therapy per protocol (e.g., increasing FIO_2 to 1.0 if not already done). Up-regulate bronchial hygiene therapy per protocol and/or add Aerosolized Medication Protocol (e.g., 2 cc 10% acetylcysteine with 0.5 cc albuterol in-line q4h). Obtain sputum for Gram stain and culture. Monitor and reevaluate.

DISCUSSION

Respiratory care of the near-drowning victim divides itself into initial and supportive care. The *initial assessment* should determine that no foreign material is obstructing the upper airway and that voluntary ventilatory efforts are being made by the patient. In this case both these items were assessed and cared for in the field, and mechanical ventilation had been started.

The second phase of management of the near-drowning victim consists of intelligent management of the ventilator, which is used first to treat the pulmonary edema that almost always accompanies the near-drowning episode and is used later to provide support during the often ensuing adult respiratory distress syndrome (ARDS)-like picture. This case demonstrates all these facets of near drowning.

In the **first assessment** the patient is inadequately ventilated and oxygenated, and the ventilator settings have not been modified to include positive end-expiratory pressure (PEEP). All these steps certainly are indicated. Vigorous tracheobronchial suctioning should be performed. The practitioner's observation of dullness to percussion and crackles **(atelectasis)** at the bases suggests that pulmonary edema **(increased alveolar-capillary membrane)** is occurring, as do the bilateral patchy infiltrates noted (see Figs. 1-8 and 1-10). Some physicians already would have performed bronchoscopy on this patient to ensure that no foreign material was in the airways.

In the **second assessment** the patient is being over-mechanically ventilated. Switching him to intermittent mandatory ventilation (IMV) mode might be wise to prevent the alveolar hyperventilation that is clearly occurring. Further adjustment of the ventilator to improve his oxygenation by an increase in the FIO_2 is indicated, as may be an increase in the ventilator PEEP setting. The patient now has frothy, white sputum, and vigorous bronchial hygiene certainly is indicated.

In the **last assessment** the patient has tachycardia, rapid respiratory rate, and core temperature elevation to 39.5° C (103° F). This indicates either central nervous system (CNS) damage or pulmonary infection. The therapist now should move quickly to assess for infection with a sputum Gram stain and culture, despite the secretions themselves being mostly frothy, pinkish-white in cases of pulmonary edema. The patient is still hypoxemic, and his blood gases are beginning to look more and more like ARDS. If the patient is already on 100% oxygen, alternative forms of mechanical ventilation, such as inverse ratio ventilation, might be considered. High PEEP pressures may be necessary, as may high mean airway pressures, and the alert therapist should have recognized this potential and had material at hand for emergency chest tube placement.

The patient died 2 days after admission. The family refused the request for an autopsy.

Chapter 28　　*Smoke Inhalation and Thermal Injuries*

Response 1

S: N/A (patient comatose, intubated on ventilator)

O: Comatose; vital signs: BP 157/105, HR 112, no spontaneous ventilations; nasal hairs singed; inability to assess oropharynx (patient intubated orally); skin: cherry-red; frothy and sooty sputum; crackles and rhonchi over both lung fields; CXR: bilateral pulmonary infiltrates consistent with pulmonary edema; ABGs: pH 7.52, $PaCO_2$ 28, HCO_3^- 22, PaO_2 202; COHb 30%; SpO_2 98%

A: • Smoke inhalation with extensive body burns
　　• Pulmonary edema (CXR, frothy sputum)
　　• Carbon monoxide poisoning (COHb 30%)
　　　　Impaired oxygen transport system
　　• Acute ventilator-induced alveolar hyperventilation with excessively corrected hypoxemia; SpO_2 misleading because of COHb (ABGs, COHb)
　　　　Excessive mechanical ventilation

P: Up-regulate Hyperinflation Therapy Protocol (e.g., increasing PEEP to 10 cm H_2O). Perform Bronchial Hygiene Therapy Protocol (e.g., suctioning frequently). Adjust Mechanical Ventilation Protocol to correct acute alveolar hyperventilation (e.g., decreasing tidal volume or rate to retain more CO_2). Continue oxygen therapy per protocol until COHb is reduced. Contact physician to consider hyperbaric oxygen (HBO) treatments and diagnostic/therapeutic bronchoscopy. Monitor and reevaluate (e.g., checking ABGs in 30 minutes).

Response 2

S: N/A (patient comatose, intubated on ventilator)

O: Skin: still cherry-red; vital signs: BP 127/88, HR 82, RR on A/C ventilation 30/min; afebrile; hemodynamics: PWCP 20 cm H_2O; frothy, sooty bronchial secretions; crackles and rhonchi auscultated over both lung fields worsening; CXR: good endotracheal tube placement, pulmonary infiltrates worsening; ABGs: pH 7.29, $PaCO_2$ 37, HCO_3^- 18, PaO_2 63; COHb 20%

A: • Pulmonary edema (CXR, frothy sputum)
　　• Carbon monoxide poisoning (COHb 20%)
　　　　Impaired oxygen transport system
　　• Metabolic acidosis with moderate hypoxemia (ABGs and COHb)

P: Continue Mechanical Ventilation Protocol. Consider sedation, paralysis, and CMV. Up-regulate hyperinflation therapy per protocol (e.g., increasing PEEP to 20 cm H_2O). Up-regulate Bronchial Hygiene Therapy Protocol (e.g., adding 2 cc 10% acetylcysteine to inline med. neb. q4h × 48 hours, trying ultrasonic nebulizer [USN], obtaining sputum Gram stain and culture). Up-regulate oxygen therapy per protocol (if possible). Discuss with doctor a re-dive in HBO until COHb <5%. Monitor and reevaluate (e.g., checking ABGs in 30 minutes).

Response 3

S: N/A (conscious but sedated; intubated, and on mechanical ventilation)

O: Excessive thick, gray and yellow secretions; sputum culture: *pseudomonas;* CXR: greater opacity throughout both lung fields, severe pulmonary edema, atelectasis, and ARDS; bronchoscopy: numerous eschars and mucus plugs suctioned; skin: no longer red; hemodynamics: normal; ABGs: pH 7.25, $Paco_2$ 39, HCO_3^- 18, Pao_2 37; COHb 10%

A: • Pulmonary edema, atelectasis, and ARDS (CXR)
  • Carbon monoxide poisoning improving (COHb 10%)
  • Metabolic acidosis with severe hypoxemia worsening (ABGs)

P: Up-regulate hyperinflation therapy per protocol (if possible). Continue bronchial hygiene therapy per protocol. Up-regulate oxygen therapy per protocol (if possible). Contact physician to consider repeat therapeutic bronchoscopy. Assist in transferring patient for HBO treatment. Monitor and reevaluate (e.g., q1-2h).

DISCUSSION

The patient with smoke inhalation or thermal injuries of the lung is a great challenge to the respiratory care professional. Initially, attention must be given to the upper airway, where one must ascertain whether the airway is obstructed by edema secondary to the thermal burn, by the burn itself, or by foreign material obstructing the airway. Once this information is known and the patient is intubated, careful respiratory care is mandatory because severe thermal injuries to the lung are usual in most such patients, and in many of them ARDS develops.

In the **first assessment** a careful examination of the upper airway is necessary. The reader should conclude that the cherry-red skin and severe carboxyhemoglobinemia are related and may account for the persistence of the patient's comatose state even after he has been intubated and placed on a ventilator. In the first assessment the patient appears to be hyperoxygenated and hyperventilated. His pulse oximeter is giving falsely high values, not correcting for the carboxyhemoglobinemia. The therapist's suggestion to increase positive end-expiratory pressure (PEEP) or the Fio_2 or both and to reduce the assist/control rate or tidal volume or both on the ventilator are appropriate. Arrangements should be made to have this patient taken to the hyperbaric oxygen (HBO) therapy unit as soon as possible, given the dangerously high carbon monoxide levels noted. Mechanical ventilation will need to be continued while he is in the HBO chamber. The fact that the patient has sooty-appearing sputum almost certainly indicates that the airway and lungs have severe thermal burns. This suspicion is confirmed by the pulmonary edema–like pattern seen on the chest x-ray.

At the **second assessment** the alert reader should conclude that the patient's acid-base status is worse, with metabolic acidosis as well as mild hypoxemia. The patient's carboxyhemoglobinemia, although improved, is still clearly an issue. The suggestion to repeat HBO therapy is appropriate. If the reader recalls that the patient's sputum culture has not yet been obtained, he or she is absolutely correct, and ordering it is appropriate. Mucolytics must be administered cautiously in this setting because a substance such as acetylcysteine may further irritate or burn the already inflamed airway. Because of this concern, 10% acetylcysteine (Mucomyst) rather than the more commonly used 20% solution is recommended. A trial of in-line ultrasonic nebulizer (USN) therapy may soothe the airway and liquefy secretions just as well.

The **last assessment** confirms that obtaining of a culture was well worthwhile because *Pseudomonas* organisms were identified. These will be treated appropriately with intravenous antibiotics. A trial of aerosolized tobramycin might be considered, to prevent the renal toxicity of the systemic use of aminoglycoside drugs. That the pulmonary edema is not clearing and the pulmonary capillary wedge pressure (PCWP) is normal suggests that the patient is developing adult respiratory distress syndrome (ARDS), which should suggest to the therapist that treatment of this patient may be prolonged. Vigorous bronchial hygiene needs to continue because eschars and mucus plugs were removed at bronchoscopy. Therapeutic bronchoscopy may be indicated repeatedly in the future. The patient continues to have metabolic acidemia, the exact cause of which should be ascertained. Because the patient's PaO_2 is so low, a repeat of HBO therapy is indicated, despite the patient's falling below the traditional COHb cutoff line of 10%.

The patient died 10 days after admission.

Chapter 29 Postoperative Atelectasis

Response 1

S: "My gut really hurts, and I can't seem to get any air."

O: Respiratory distress; cyanosis; vital signs: BP 185/90, HR 130, RR 35, T normal; tachypnea; frequent spontaneous, weak cough with yellow sputum production; LLL: diminished breath sounds; RLL: bronchial breath sounds and dull percussion notes; incentive spirometry (IS): 40% preoperative value; SpO_2 (2 L/min O_2 by nasal cannula) 77%; ABGs: pH 7.57, $PaCO_2$ 23, HCO_3^- 21, PaO_2 43; poor cooperation with IS

A: • Labored breathing (general appearance, vital signs, ABGs)
 • Excessive yellow sputum accumulation (sputum)
  Possible infection
 • Weak cough effort (observation)
 • Possible atelectasis or consolidation or both in RLL (dull percussion, bronchial breath sound, IS values)
 • Acute alveolar hyperventilation with moderate-to-severe hypoxemia (ABGs)
 • Poor patient cooperation with IS

P: Initiate Oxygen Therapy Protocol (e.g., O_2 via HAFOE mask with FIO_2 0.60). Begin Bronchial Hygiene Therapy Protocol (e.g., CPT and nasotracheal suction q4h and prn; sputum for culture). Begin Hyperinflation Therapy Protocol (e.g., face CPAP mask at 10 cm H_2O × 5 minutes q2h while awake). Administer Aerosolized Medication Protocol (e.g., med. nebs. with 0.5 cc albuterol in 2 cc 20% acetylcysteine q4h). Request chest x-ray film. Monitor and reevaluate (e.g., checking ABGs in 30 minutes).

Response 2

S: No response to questions

O: Respiratory distress: cyanotic, cool, and damp skin; vital signs: BP 188/100, HR 135, RR 36, T 38.1° C (100.6° F); right middle and both lower lung lobes: dull percussion notes, bronchial breath sounds, and crackles; CXR: RML, RLL, and LLL atelectasis and air bronchograms; SpO_2 72%; ABGs: pH 7.55, $PaCO_2$ 29, HCO_3^- 22, PaO_2 46

A: • Continued labored breathing (general appearance, vital signs, ABGs)
 • Sputum accumulation still excessive (cough and recent history)
 • Weak cough effort (observation)
 • RML, RLL, and LLL atelectasis (CXR, dull percussion, bronchial breath sounds)
 • Acute alveolar hyperventilation with moderate-to-severe hypoxemia (ABGs)
  Impending ventilatory failure

P: Call doctor stat and request transfer to ICU. Up-regulate oxygen therapy per protocol (e.g., increasing FIO_2 to 0.80). Up-regulate bronchial hygiene therapy per protocol (e.g., increasing CPT to q2h). Up-regulate hyperinflation therapy per protocol (e.g., increasing CPAP mask to 15 cm H_2O). Up-regulate aerosolized medication therapy per protocol (e.g., increasing med. nebs. to q2h). Continue to monitor and evaluate closely.

Response 3

S: "I think I'm dying."

O: Obvious respiratory distress; skin cyanotic, cool, and damp; no right-sided chest excursion; trachea deviated to the right; vital signs: BP 192/90, HR 142, RR 20, T 37.3° C (99.1° F); RML and RLL: bronchial breath sounds, crackles, and dull percussion notes; LLL: dull percussion notes and no breath sounds; SpO_2 62%; ABGs: pH 7.26, $PaCO_2$ 53, HCO_3^- 22, PaO_2 37

A: • Continued increased work of breathing (general appearance, vital signs)
- Excessive sputum accumulation still likely (recent history)
- RML and RLL atelectasis (dull percussion, bronchial breath sounds, CXR)
- Possible LLL atelectasis (dull percussion note, CXR)
   Likely caused by mucus plugging (no breath sounds)
- Acute ventilatory failure with severe hypoxemia (ABGs)

P: Contact physician stat. Recommend intubation and mechanical ventilation accompanied by the following: oxygen therapy per protocol, bronchial hygiene therapy per protocol, hyperinflation therapy per protocol, and aerosolized medication therapy per protocol.

DISCUSSION

By the time of the **first assessment** this overweight, tobacco-abusing woman with a chronic productive cough *before* surgery has developed postoperative atelectasis due to pain, splinting of the chest, or postoperative analgesia. The physical findings are classic for major atelectasis initially involving the right lung and associated with severe right-to-left shunt physiology, despite alveolar hyperventilation.

In the first portion of this case the diagnosis and treatment of postoperative atelectasis with incentive spirometry (IS; and failing that, intermittent positive-pressure breathing [IPPB]) is fairly straightforward. The patient's severe hypoxemia, despite alveolar hyperventilation, however, deserves careful monitoring. Giving this patient a much higher concentration of oxygen (e.g., 50%) by a Venturi oxygen mask is probably safe. However, careful attention must be paid to oximetry and blood gas analyses. If the patient did not wake up and become more cooperative at this point, the blood gases are severe enough to prompt consideration of intubation and mechanical ventilation at this time.

If one "SOAPs" this patient carefully, a heavy preoperative cigarette smoking history should be noted. The alert reader would have started bronchial hygiene therapy per protocol. The mild diastolic hypertension, which has persisted despite analgesia, is worrisome and needs to be monitored carefully.

At the time of the **second assessment** the patient will not or could not cooperate with deep breathing and coughing and categorically refused chest physical therapy. The blood pressure is even higher; the heart rate is rapid; and the patient has a fever as well. That the patient is unresponsive raises the question of sedation overdose and possible CO_2 retention, but the blood gases clearly rule out CO_2 retention.

Based on the physical findings and chest x-ray film the therapist appropriately assesses the cause as right middle and lower lobe atelectasis and possible left lower lobe atelectasis. Oxygen therapy is pushed correctly with an increase in the F_{IO_2} by mask therapy. However, because of the right-to-left shunt physiology involved, this result may not be successful. Bronchial hygiene and aerosolized medication therapy per protocols are indicated as well, with vigorous bronchodilation, mucolysis, and consideration of therapeutic bronchoscopy. The patient's arterial blood gases are abnormal enough to make intubation and mechanical ventilation options at this point. Sputum from deep nasotracheal suctioning or bronchoscopy should be cultured promptly because the patient's fever most likely represents pulmonary infection.

Certainly at the **final assessment** the patient must be mechanically ventilated; she has acute respiratory acidosis and profound hypoxemia. Her bilateral atelectasis is still present and has not been improved by the treatments outlined previously. By the time of the *final assessment* the patient has gone beyond the usual medical boundaries. The treating therapist's desire to contact the physician immediately and prepare for semiemergent mechanical ventilation is entirely appropriate. Inflation therapy with positive end-expiratory pressure (PEEP) as part of the mechanical ventilation order also would be appropriate because atelectasis clearly is the chief villain.

Despite vigorous therapy as outlined in this case, the patient did poorly. After 5 days, she was able to be weaned gradually from ventilator support and after 2 weeks, she was able to return home. Postoperative infection and retained secretions characterized her postoperative course. As of her last follow-up visit, she continued to smoke, despite advice to the contrary. Return demonstrations of IS and appropriate metered dose inhaler (MDI) use were never satisfactory in the course of her hospitalization.

KEY POINT ANSWERS

For Postoperative Atelectasis (DRG* 101/102)

1. Basic Concept Formation
   a. It becomes *smaller,* collapsed in on itself.
   b. The airless lung *could not oxygenate* blood passing through it, and hypoxemia would result.
   c. *Airway obstruction* (from mucus plugging) and *small tidal volume breathing* (as under fractured ribs).
   d. *Yes.* Effective coughing and secretion removal are key elements in both the prevention and treatment of atelectasis and are delivered as part of the Bronchial Hygiene Therapy Protocol. Hyperinflation therapy (incentive spirometry [IS], intermittent positive-pressure breathing [IPPB], positive expiratory pressure [PEP], continuous positive airway pressure [CPAP], and positive end-expiratory pressure [PEEP] administration) is also a key element in the prevention and treatment of atelectasis.
2. Database Formation
   a. Atelectatic areas of the lung are *small* and *airless.*†
   b. *Decreased* $\dot{V}/\dot{Q}$ *ratio,* producing *right-to-left shunt physiology* and *hypoxemia,* and *decreased lung compliance,* producing *restrictive lung function physiology* (see Fig. 1-8) are activated. A small lung is a noncompliant lung.
   c. *Yes.* The airway *lumen* is often obstructed, and *airless surrounding structures* do not readily transmit intrapleural distending forces to obstructed, small lung units.
   d. Eventually, *acute respiratory failure* will occur. Some evidence also supports the notion that reduced cough efficiency in such patients leads to *retained secretions* and possibly to pneumonia. Atelectasis can be progressive, involving more and more lung parenchyma. A vicious circle—difficult-to-expand lung → retained secretions → more atelectasis → more retained secretions—develops and can lead (as in this case) to ventilatory insufficiency and ventilatory failure.
   e. Atelectasis unfortunately is a common postoperative complication. Operative site pain, chest wall splinting, air swallowing with distension of abdominal viscera, and failure to cough and deep breathe are all factors in the development of postoperative atelectasis. Basically, atelectasis also may result when an airway is obstructed from any cause, and air distal to the obstruction is absorbed into the pulmonary circulation. This process is accelerated when the P_{AO_2} is high and is sometimes called *absorption atelectasis.* Finally, alveolar hypoventilation from any cause may result in atelectasis, either regionally or throughout the lung. Thus atelectasis can occur in the following instances:
      1. Chest wall injuries (flail chest)
      2. Obesity
      3. Myasthenia gravis and Guillain-Barré syndrome
      4. Cervical spine injuries
      5. Under pleuritic areas of lung
      6. Under pneumothoraces or pleural effusions
      7. Conditions reducing pulmonary compliance, such as pulmonary fibrosis, pulmonary edema, and adult respiratory distress syndrome (ARDS)

---

*DRG, Diagnosis-related group.

†See color plate 37 in Des Jardins T, Burton GG: Clinical manifestations and assessment of respiratory disease, ed 4, St Louis, 2002, Mosby.

Continued

f. The *goals of therapy* in patients with atelectasis are to (1) remove secretions obstructing the airways, (2) induce deep breaths and sighs, (3) remove any extrinsic compressing factors, such as pleural effusion or pneumothorax, (4) maintain alveolar stability by increasing mean airway and end-expiratory pressure, and (5) oxygenate the patient.

g. *Oxygen Therapy, Hyperinflation Therapy,* and *Bronchial Hygiene Therapy Protocols* are indicated in all patients with hypoxemia resulting from excessive airway secretions and atelectasis. The Aerosolized Medication Protocol to deliver bronchodilators and/or mucolytics also may be used if airway obstruction from bronchospasm and/or retained secretions are observed.

1. *Potential adverse effects* of these protocols include the following:
   a. *Oxygen therapy:* absorption atelectasis (see answer 2.e) and (remotely possible) cellular oxygen toxicity
   b. *Hyperinflation therapy* (especially with IPPB and PEEP): pulmonary barotrauma
   c. *Bronchial hygiene:* no specific adverse effects
   d. *Aerosolized Medication:* toxicity related to the aerosolized medication(s) being used (e.g., tachycardia from beta$_2$ stimulants; airway irritation from acetylcysteine)

2. Appropriate monitors in atelectasis include serial inspiratory capacity (IC) or forced vital capacity (FVC) measurements, *pulse oximetry,* and arterial blood gas values (ABGs); with calculation of A-a O$_2$ gradient or PaO_2/FIO_2 ratio), *serial chest x-ray,* and in intubated, mechanically ventilated patients, serial measurement of *static pulmonary compliance.*

3. Assessment
   a. *Yes.* Her smoking history, obesity, current history of pneumonia, asthma, chronic obstructive pulmonary disease (COPD), the site of surgery, and the length of the procedure all predispose a patient to the development of postoperative atelectasis.
   b. *Yes.* She demonstrated tachycardia and tachypnea, hypertension, findings of consolidation (dullness to percussion, bronchial breath sounds) in the right lower lobe, restrictive physiology on pulmonary function testing, and hypoxemia, all *expected clinical manifestations of atelectasis* (see Fig. 1-8). The presence of crackles over the RML and RLL in the *second* assessment suggest alveolar consolidation or atelectasis. Both pneumonia and atelectasis may be the cause when crackles are heard on auscultation.
   c. *Yes.* Her *shunt physiology* was reflected in oxygen-refractory hypoxemia. Her *reduced pulmonary compliance* was reflected in her rapid, shallow breathing, restrictive pulmonary function test results, and chest x-ray film.
   d. Following are the clinical manifestations that indicated the severity of the condition:
      1. On the *first* assessment her cyanosis, tachypnea, fall in FVC to 40% of preoperative volumes, and severe hypoxemia despite low-flow oxygen therapy and hyperventilation all indicate the *seriousness* of her situation.
      2. On the *second* assessment she is unresponsive, still tachypneic, and hypoxemic. These findings indicate *worsening,* as her comatose condition precludes use of incentive spirometry. Her hypoxemia could worsen *further* if, for example, "heavy-duty" analgesia, such as morphine sulfate, were given; her pain were relieved; and her pain-mediated hyperventilation were to cease.

3. On the *third and last* assessment the patient has slipped into acute respiratory failure, with respiratory acidemia and even worse ABGs.

4. Application
   a. Sputum induction *was not* indicated, although she had been producing yellow sputum that had not previously been cultured. If the patient is coughing productively, no need exists to induce sputum. The respiratory care practitioner was correct in sending a specimen off to the laboratory because infection (bronchitis or pneumonia) can cause atelectasis.
   b. Oxygen therapy certainly *was* indicated because of her hypoxemia.
   c. Bronchial hygiene therapy *was* indicated because of her smoking history, history of productive cough, and bronchial breath sounds. Airway secretions often obstruct airways and lead to atelectasis (see answer 1.c). Their prompt expectoration or removal by coughing or suctioning both prevent and treat atelectasis. Such is the rationale for deep breathing and coughing (C&DB), percussion and postural drainage (PD), and therapeutic bronchoscopy.
   d. Hyperinflation therapy certainly *was* indicated and is the core of prevention and treatment of postoperative atelectasis.
   e. Aerosolized medication therapy *was* indicated, at least on a trial basis, because of the patient's smoking history and sputum production at the time of the first assessment.
   f. At the time of the last assessment, *mechanical ventilation was* indicated because of her severely abnormal ABGs.
   g. When the patient recovered, *pulmonary rehabilitation was* indicated for smoking-cessation education and use of inhaled bronchodilators alone, if for no other reason. *Summary of need for therapy:* Note in this patient indications for multiple therapeutic modalities. The reader should contrast this finding with the needs of the patient with simple pneumonia, whose chest radiograph may appear very similar to this patient's.

5. Evaluation
   a. The respiratory care practitioner can expect the following results and complications from the choice of therapeutic modalities:
      1. *Oxygen therapy:* relief of the patient's hypoxemia to the extent allowed by her shunt physiology; complications are rare
      2. *Bronchial hygiene therapy:* initially, increased volume of expectorated sputum, reduction in rhonchi, arrest of atelectasis; complications rare
      3. *Hyperinflation therapy:* increase in IC or FVC, improvement in chest x-ray and ABGs as atelectasis improves; arrest of atelectasis; periodic assessment to guide the choice between IS and IPPB therapy; IS generally being better tolerated than IPPB, and the volume-time integral being better for IS; air swallowing and barotrauma being known complications of IPPB but not of IS
      4. *Aerosolized medication therapy:* In this case, improvement in clearance of sputum, increase in IC or FVC, reduction in shunt fraction ($\dot{Q}s/\dot{Q}t$), and better blood gas values; complications of aerosolized medication therapy listed in answer 2.g, including tachycardia and irritation of the airway
      5. *Mechanical ventilation:* PEEP therapy used if hypoxemia not improved; improved respiratory acidemia; barotrauma being the feared complication of mechanical ventilation
      6. *Pulmonary rehabilitation:* Improved bronchial hygiene; importance of smoking cessation understood by the patient; increased level of day-to-day functioning, activities of daily living; complications are rare
   b. *Monitors* for the success or failure of each modality are as follows:
      1. *Oxygen therapy:* SpO_2, ABGs
      2. *Bronchial hygiene therapy:* sputum volume/type, chest x-ray, SpO_2, ABGs

Continued

KEY POINT ANSWERS—cont'd

   3. *Hyperinflation therapy:* IC, FVC, SpO_2, ABGs, chest x-ray film
   4. *Aerosolized medication therapy:* FVC, ABGs, sputum volume and viscosity, chest x-ray clearance, improved static compliance (if patient on mechanical ventilator)
   5. *Mechanical ventilation:* ABGs, SpO_2, static compliance

c. The *upper limits* of intensity or frequency of the necessary modalities are as follows:
   1. *Oxygen therapy:* This modality can be increased to an FIO_2 of 1.0.
   2. *Bronchial hygiene therapy:* Deep breathing and coughing instruction or exercises can practically be done every 30 to 60 minutes. Percussion and PD are not tolerated more often than once every 2 to 3 hours. Therapeutic bronchoscopy can be done as often as necessary, although it usually is accompanied by intubation after the second or third procedure.
   3. *Hyperinflation therapy:* IS or IPPB or both can be done initially every 30 to 60 minutes. IPPB is not indicated if the patient will not or cannot use IS, if the chest x-ray film documents increasing atelectasis, if C&DB and IS are unsuccessful in preventing or treating atelectasis, or if the IC is <30% of predicted normal values. PEP, CPAP, and PEEP can be done continuously.
   4. *Aerosolized medication therapy:* This modality can be increased practically, every 2 to 3 hours without undue side effects.
   5. *Mechanical Ventilation:* This modality is done continuously. Barotrauma limits therapy.

d. The *least invasive* of the indicated therapies for atelectasis are C&DB, IS, aerosolized medications, mask CPAP, and O_2 therapy. *More intrusive* are IPPB and bronchodilation therapy. *More expensive and invasive* and associated with known side effects or risks are therapeutic bronchoscopy, mechanical ventilation, and PEEP therapy. Despite this hierarchy of risks and costs, early use of therapeutic bronchoscopy often is ultimately cost effective because it treats atelectasis secondary to airway obstruction at its core.

e. If the monitors listed in answer 5.b indicate *improvement,* discontinue mechanical ventilation and extubate the patient first, maintaining aggressive bronchial hygiene, aerosolized medication, and hyperinflation therapy in the form of IS for at least 3 to 4 days thereafter. Oxygen therapy should be tapered as ABGs or SpO_2 volumes allow.

f. If the patient *does not improve* (as in this case), aggressive therapeutic bronchoscopy, intubation, and mechanical ventilation with pressure support and PEEP are indicated.

6. Boundary Awareness
a. This patient is critically ill at the time of the *first* assessment (see answer 3.d) and progressively worsens in the next two scenarios. Her ABGs, SpO_2 values, and chest x-ray films all point to this.

b. Ask a supervisor for help literally at *any time* in the case of this critically ill patient, certainly at the time of the *third* assessment.

c. As in answer 6.b, call the physician at any time in this case. In cases of atelectasis, the suggestion is that a physician be called when the SpO_2 cannot be kept above 88%, when respiratory or metabolic acidosis supravenes, when a new lobe collapses on the chest x-ray film, and whenever bronchoscopy or mechanical ventilation appears necessary.

SOAP Form

Respiratory Assessment Flow Chart

Subjective →

Objective →

Vital signs: RR ______ HR ______ BP ______

Temp. ______ On antipyretic agent? ☐ Yes ☐ No

Chest assessment:

Insp. ______

Palp. ______

Perc. ______

Ausc. ______

Radiography ______

Bedside spir.: PEFR ā ______ p̄ ______ Tx

SVC ______ FVC ______ NIF ______

Cough: ☐ Strong ☐ Weak

Sputum production: ☐ Yes ☐ No

Sputum char. ______

ABG: pH ______ $Paco_2$ ______ HCO_3^- ______

Pao_2 ______ Sao_2 ______ Spo_2 ______

Neg. O_2 transport factors ______

Other: ______

Assessment →

Plan →

Present Plan

Plan Modifications

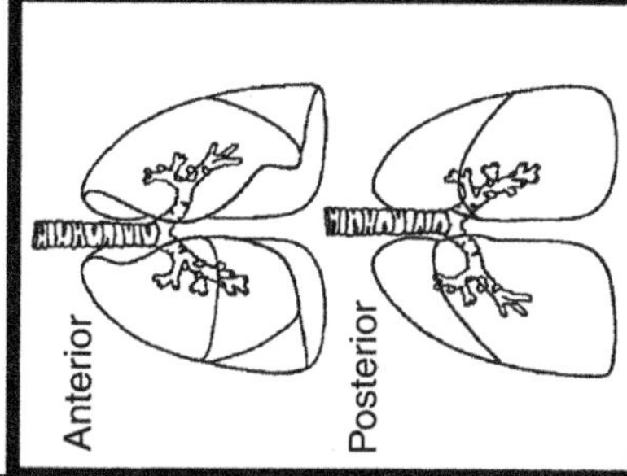

Anterior
Posterior

Pt. name		
Age	Male	Female
Date	Time	
Admitting diagnosis		
Therapist		
Hospital		

Index

Italic page numbers indicate illustrations; t indicates a table.

Printed and bound by CPI Group (UK) Ltd, Croydon, CR0 4YY

03/10/2024

01040364-0010